DAOIST MERIDIAN YOGA

of related interest

Fire Dragon Meridian Qigong
Essential NeiGong for Health and Spiritual Transformation
Master Zhongxian Wu and Dr Karin Taylor Wu
ISBN 978 1 84819 103 7
eISBN 978 0 85701 085 8

The Four Dragons
Clearing the Meridians and Awakening the Spine in Nei Gong
Damo Mitchell
Foreword by Dr Ole Saether
ISBN 978 1 84819 226 3
eISBN 978 0 85701 173 2

Qigong Through the Seasons
How to Stay Healthy All Year with Qigong, Meditation, Diet, and Herbs
Ronald H. Davis
Illustrated by Pamm Davis
Foreword by Ken Cohen
ISBN 978 1 84819 238 6
eISBN 978 0 85701 185 5

The Way of the Five Elements
52 weeks of powerful acupoints for physical, emotional, and spiritual health
John Kirkwood
ISBN 978 1 84819 270 6
eISBN 978 0 85701 216 6

DAOIST MERIDIAN YOGA

ACTIVATING THE TWELVE PATHWAYS FOR ENERGY BALANCE AND HEALING

Camilo Sanchez, L.Ac., MOM

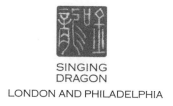

SINGING
DRAGON
LONDON AND PHILADELPHIA

The channel diagrams at the beginnings of Chapters 4–15 have been reproduced from https://manumissio.wikispaces.com in accordance with the Creative Commons License 3.0.

First published in 2016
by Singing Dragon
an imprint of Jessica Kingsley Publishers
73 Collier Street
London N1 9BE, UK
and
400 Market Street, Suite 400
Philadelphia, PA 19106, USA

www.singingdragon.com

Copyright © Camilo Sanchez, L.Ac., MOM 2016
Photography: Jasiatic

Library of Congress Cataloging in Publication Data
A CIP catalog record for this book is available from the Library of Congress

British Library Cataloguing in Publication Data
A CIP catalogue record for this book is available from the British Library

ISBN 978 1 84819 285 0
eISBN 978 0 85701 236 4

Printed and bound in Great Britain

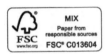

I want to dedicate this instructional guide to my Guru Paramahansa Swami Satyananda, who revealed the genuine nature of Yoga and Tantra; my teacher Reverend Dr. Richard Browne, who initiated me into the Daoist healing arts and spiritual healing; Shifu Frank Paolillo, for generously imparting the true teachings of the Dao tradition and Taiji; and my teacher Master Zhang Xue-Xin, for transmitting the essence of Qigong and internal martial arts.

DISCLAIMER

The information provided in this book is written solely for educational and recreational purposes. The author and publishers of this book are not liable or responsible whatsoever for any loss, damage, or injury resulting directly or indirectly from following the instructions, exercises, advice, or performances presented in this book. The activities and exercises presented in this book may be too strenuous, difficult, or risky for some people and not suitable for everyone. As with any physical exercise there is always the risk of injury. Before engaging in this or any exercise program or physical activity it is recommended that you consult with your doctor or primary health provider. Other special cautions may apply to individuals with specific health issues. The advice and information provided in this book is not intended to diagnose, treat, cure, or prevent any disease or medical condition or as a substitute for professional medical care. Please, always use caution when engaging in any exercise program.

CONTENTS

PREFACE

The system of Daoist Meridian Yoga was developed from studies, research and practice of yoga, Chinese medicine and *Qigong* carried out for over 25 years.

I first trained in yoga at the Satyananda ashram of Munger, India, where I lived as a sannyasin (monastic) between 1982 and 1985. At the ashram we didn't have any "formal training" in yoga, in the sense of taking regular yoga classes. It was a lifestyle. We learned yoga by living the yogic way of life. What unfolded while living at the ashram was a process of inner purification; the physical body was purified through wholesome vegetarian food and the cleansing practices of hatha yoga, the mind underwent purification by being actively engaged and focused on the tasks at hand and minimizing external distractions like radio, television, reading, newspapers, and even unnecessary conversation, and the heart was purified through selfless service without expectations. At the same time, the whole atmosphere at the ashram was somehow conducive to this process of inner purification as the foundation for the higher meditative practices and kriyas of yoga. It was a dynamic, mindful and service-oriented lifestyle at the ashram. Swami Satyananda was of the opinion that the mind and vital energy should first be expressed and extroverted before they are brought inward in meditation. Cultivating an active and dynamic attitude allows the contents of the subconscious mind to be expressed and released so as to unravel and liberate the habitual patterns of energy and consciousness ingrained in the deeper layers of the mind. Actually, by casting-out and releasing the veil of past impressions, the mind will naturally achieve stillness and clarity.

We did receive yoga instruction about teaching yoga as a holistic, comprehensive and systematic approach to physical and spiritual development, and also underwent training on the six purifications techniques of hatha yoga, utilized to cleanse the upper respiratory system, digestive system and elimination system, as the ashram conducted regular yoga classes and sadhana (spiritual practice) intensive courses for the public. At the same time, we were exposed to the deeper dimensions of yoga practice. In this manner, while living at the ashram we learned the science of yoga through inner receptivity and direct transmission.

I remember one occasion that a sannyasin resident at the ashram asked our Guru Swami Satyananda why we didn't have more regular yoga classes at the ashram. Swami Satyananda explained that people living in society needed yoga practice to counteract the imbalances and pressures of daily living. For them, regular yoga techniques provided a potent and excellent means to remedy the stresses of modern living, release tension, regain vitality and balance the mind. He further said that sannyasins at the ashram lived a simple, dynamic, highly aware and natural yogic lifestyle so didn't need a lot of yoga practice. At the same time, Swami Satyananda presented yoga as a holistic and comprehensive science for harmonizing the physical, emotional and spiritual aspects of the human personality, and as a practice suitable for every walk of life.

Later on, in 1986 I came to the States to study Chinese medicine and acupuncture at the Acupuncture and Massage College in Miami, Florida. As I learned Chinese medicine, in particular the system of acupuncture energy meridians or channels, I began to have a better understanding of many of the yoga techniques I was exposed to during my stay at the ashram and how these yoga practices affected the physiologic functions and the various subtle energies, channels, centers, and vital points of the body. At the same time, I was also initiated in the Chinese practices of *Taiji* and Daoist *Qigong*.

After graduating from the Acupuncture and Massage College, I joined the school's faculty and began teaching Chinese medicine. It is said that if one really wants to learn something in depth one should teach it. In fact, teaching all areas of Chinese medicine, as well as supervising the community acupuncture clinic at the school and running my own private acupuncture practice, gave me the opportunity to dive down and deeply study Chinese medicine, enhancing my understanding of the system of the energy meridians.

Over the next 15 years I studied, practiced, and researched various methods of Chinese *Qigong* with notable teachers including George Xu, Wei Zhong Foo, Frank Chang, Sifu Frank Paolillo, Chunyi Lin, Master Zhang Xue-Xin, Shu Dong Li, and Feng Wang Ming, among others. At the same time, I continued my studies of Chen style *Taiji* and *Bagua*. It was during this time that I began revising and synthesizing the various Daoist *Qigong* exercises based on their action upon the twelve primary acupuncture meridians. I also started teaching the first version of the 24 exercises at weekly classes and weekend seminars. The exercises were fine-tuned and refined over twelve years based on my ongoing personal practice and the experience and feedback of students and patients alike, until they reached the present format.

I am happy to present this system of Daoist Meridian Yoga exercises to practitioners, students, and enthusiasts of Chinese medicine, *Qigong*, yoga, and the healing and movement arts, as well as to the general public. It is my hope that it will provide you with a complete meridian workout, overall Qi balancing and self-healing practice.

Lao Shi Camilo Sanchez, L.Ac., MOM
Charlotte, NC
August 26, 2015

Introduction

The Chinese medicine model of healing

The system of Daoist Meridian Yoga exercises is based on the greater traditions of *Qigong, Daoyin,* and Chinese medicine. Here we provide a brief introduction to *Qigong* and the Chinese medicine model of healing.

Chinese medicine is a comprehensive system of healing that has been practiced uninterruptedly for over 2500 years. Even today, it is still the preferred form of health care for over half the world population. Traditionally, Chinese medicine comprised eight main branches that included Chinese herbal medicine, acupuncture, Chinese massage (*anmo*), nutrition, Daoist cosmology and philosophy, *Feng Shui* (balance of the living environment), *Qigong* (energy exercises), and meditation.

Qigong is a generic term for the various practices of cultivating the vital energy or Qi. The term *Qigong* is comprised of two Chinese characters: *Qi* means the innate vital life energy within the body with which we are endowed from before birth; *Gong* refers to a skill, attainment, or mastery obtained over time through regular practice. Thus, together, the term *Qigong* means the practice and mastery of Qi or internal life energy.

Qigong exercises have a long tradition of practice that developed from centuries of experimentation, study, and research. In ancient times *Qigong* exercises were known by various names such as *Daoyin* (stretching the body and guiding Qi), *Xing Qi* (circulating Qi), *Tu Na* (exhaling and inhaling exercises), *Fu Qi* (taking Qi), *An Qiao* (energy massage), and *Shi Qi* (living on Qi), among others.

Qi is the vital essence and intelligence that drives the functioning of the body. Our life energy, stamina, vitality, immunity, health, enthusiasm, and even mental condition are directly dependent on the state of our Qi. Therefore, in the Chinese model of medicine, cultivating and strengthening our Qi is the most essential principle for improving our health.

The practice of *Qigong* consists of a combination of slow and flowing movements, breathing techniques, mind focus, and guiding vital energy or Qi. The various techniques of *Qigong* can be used to unlock, harness, strengthen, circulate, and refine the body's internal energy or Qi in order to enhance and optimize the function and performance of the body and mind. Thus, from early times the healing modalities of Chinese medicine and *Qigong* were integrated into a holistic system of health.

Qigong and Daoist yoga exercises are gaining popularity and becoming better known in the West as a mind–body practice for maintaining high levels of health, promoting self-healing, treating and preventing disease, boosting vitality, delaying premature aging, and developing the potential abilities of the human body and mind.

In the traditions of Chinese medicine and *Qigong*, central to the understanding of the human body, is the notion of vital life energy or Qi. In the view of Chinese medicine, life is the result of the interplay between the opposite and complementary energies of Yin and Yang. The whirling of galaxies, orbiting of planets, and the ever-changing cycle of the seasons all show us the workings of the life force in the natural world. Similarly, in the human body, vital energy or Qi manifests as the various physiologic functions from the blink of an eye to a heartbeat and general metabolism.

According to *Qigong* and Chinese medicine the human being is a combination of body (*Jing*), vital energy (*Qi*), and spirit or consciousness (*Shen*). Spirit directs vital energy, vital energy activates the body, and the body is the carrier of both energy and spirit. Thus, *Jing* makes up the most substantial or condensed form of energy, *Qi* comprises our refined or subtle energy which acts as the motive force for the functions of the body, and *Shen* is considered a high-level energy that controls the information of both the body and vital energy.

Modern physics tells us that the core of matter is energy, and ultimately solid matter is frozen or condensed light. Energy is described as the potential to cause change and it manifests by its effects. Likewise, Chinese medicine and *Qigong* view the body as comprised of vital energy centers (*Dantian*), energy channels (*Jing Luo*), and energy points (*Qi Xue*).

The nature of the energy meridians

The human body has a complex system of nerve pathways and blood vessels that carry nerve signals and transport nutritive elements to coordinate and nourish the various tissues and functions of the organism. In the same way, there is an intricate network of energy channels or meridians that transmit vital energy signals and information throughout the body. The system of energy meridians includes superficial, intermediate, and deep energy pathways. The superficial pathways run along the surface of the skin and superficial tissues, while the internal branches run deep and connect with the internal organs and tissues of the body. There are also connecting or collateral channels that link the primary channels. The vital energy points are located along the external path of the meridian and are commonly depicted on acupuncture charts.

The energy centers (*Dantian*) act like focal points and reservoirs that store and produce vital energy. In turn, the meridians are the main pathways for the distribution of vital energy in the body. The energy meridians are not just flat lines that run longitudinally up and down the body; rather, we should understand the meridians as magnetic vectors and tri-dimensional energy fields that affect how vital substances, particles, and energy signals move inside the body.

In this way, the energy meridians work circulating and distributing vital energy, connecting the internal organs with the external tissues, regulating the functions of the body, and linking the various physiologic systems making the body an integrated whole.

The energy meridians and the muscle groups

As noted above, the energy meridians have external pathways along the superficial tissues of the body and are linked with specific muscle groups on the surface of the body.

According to the system of acupuncture therapy there are six types of energy pathways in the body. The most superficial pathways are the musculoskeletal or sinew channels (*Jin Jing*). They run on the surface of the body along the superficial muscles and tissues and for the most part follow the course of the primary acupuncture energy pathways.

Daoist meridian exercises involve lengthening two ends of the body in opposite directions and connecting the musculoskeletal structure, while simultaneously stretching, toning, and extending the system of fascia and connective tissue linked with the energy meridians. They work by making use of the primary action of their related muscle groups. In this way, the exercises stimulate specific vital energy points along the external pathway of the meridians. At the same time, through the opening, closing, and folding actions of the chest and abdomen, the exercises activate the deeper branches of the energy channels and important acupuncture reflex points on the trunk that directly influence the function of the internal organs. The synergistic action of these techniques along with guiding Qi to the targeted areas helps in opening, activating, and linking the flow of vital energy along the energy meridians.

In the author's clinical and teaching experience, as well as from numerous testimonies from patients and clients over the last twelve years, it has been shown that regular practice of Daoist Meridian Yoga exercises helps to stimulate circulation, improve breathing capacity, strengthen the immune system and resistance to disease, promote digestion, increase muscle tone and flexibility, increase vitality and energy level, support the healing of chronic health disorders, activate the powers of regeneration, promote optimum health, reduce stress, improve mood, and balance the mind.

I invite you to follow this comprehensive instructional guide to Daoist Meridian Yoga exercises as a regular energy practice for empowering your own health and well-being.

Part I

THE SYSTEM OF DAOIST MERIDIAN YOGA

The following chapters will introduce you to the system of Daoist Meridian Yoga and the theories behind the exercises. We will also explain the principles involved in the practice and how the exercises work.

The guide to practicing the exercises will describe four ways of performing them, thus allowing you to choose the method that best suits your needs.

So, whether you are looking for a complete Qi fitness practice or individual exercises to address specific health concerns, the system of Daoist Meridian Yoga will help awaken your power of self-healing, optimize your health, and renew your life energy.

Enjoy it!

Chapter 1

Introduction to the System of Daoist Meridian Yoga

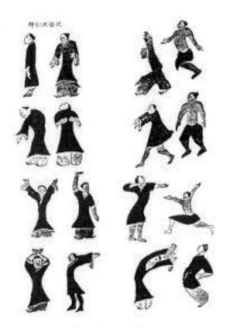

Daoyin exercises

Daoist Meridian Yoga is a system of Chinese health, preventative, and self-healing exercises based on the traditions of *Daoyin* (pulling and guiding Qi), *Qigong* (energy exercises), and principles of Chinese medicine.

Daoyin is sometimes referred to as "Chinese Yoga" and it encompasses a great variety of health exercises that focus on stretching the body and guiding the flow of Qi or vital energy. The word "yoga" is a Sanskrit term meaning "to yoke, join, bind or bring together," referring to the integration of the human personality and the union of the individual consciousness (Atman) with the universal consciousness (Brahman). While the term yoga is of Indian origin, it can be rightly used to describe the Daoist meridian exercises as they emphasize the integration of the body, vital energy, and mind, as well as cultivating a higher level of awareness.

Traditionally, *Daoyin* exercises were utilized for cultivating Qi or the vital energy of the body, improving health, and promoting longevity. In addition, they served as the foundation for refining the spirit and attuning to Dao or our original nature.

Qi: the healing power of life energy

The principle of Qi has permeated the Chinese culture for over four thousand years. Qi can have several meanings depending on the context in which it is used. Commonly, Qi is associated with air, vapor, and breath. However, in the context of Daoist yoga, Qi does not just mean the breath or air that we take in and out of the nose; rather, it refers to the innate life energy within the body. It is the inborn energy with which we are naturally endowed from birth. Accordingly, it is called "original Qi" (*Yuan Qi*) or "true Qi" (*Zhen Qi*) to differentiate it from the air we take in.

Daoist Meridian Yoga exercises work by stretching, lengthening, and toning specific muscle groups associated with the twelve energy meridians (Qi channels). The Qi channels are integrated and interact with the system of muscles, fascia, tendons, ligaments, bones, and internal organs into a network that extends throughout the body. It is estimated that Qi flows through the fibrous system of fascia and connective tissue that wraps, binds and supports the various structures and internal organs of the body into a unified whole. Thus, linking, lengthening, and stretching the system of fascia and connective tissue helps to open and activate the flow of internal Qi through the energy meridians.

Moreover, enlivening and opening up the flow of internal energy is the master key for awakening the healing potential of the human body and mind.

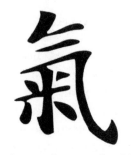

Chinese character for Qi

The system of energy meridians

Note: The energy meridians are also known as the Qi channels. In this book the two terms are used interchangeably.

A fundamental notion of the Daoist experience is that humanity is placed between heaven and earth. Heaven is the source of *Yang Qi* (the creative and active energy) and earth is the root of *Yin Qi* (the receptive and nurturing energy). Thus, the human body acts as a vessel for the interplay of these two great forces of nature.

In Chinese medicine the anatomical position of the human body is standing with the arms extended above the head, the palms facing the front, and the feet deeply rooted on the earth. In this position of the body *Yang Qi* flows from the hands and head down the back of the body and along the posterior aspect of the extremities to the feet. In turn, *Yin Qi* flows from the feet up the front of the body to the abdomen and chest and along the anterior aspect of the extremities to the hands.

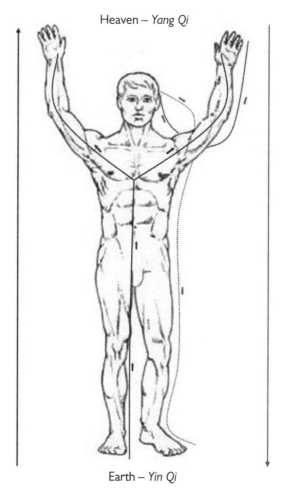

Heaven – *Yang Qi*

Earth – *Yin Qi*

The flow of *Yang Qi* and *Yin Qi* in the body

Yang and Yin channels

Yang Qi channels: posterior aspect of the body

Hands → Head → Feet

Yin Qi channels: anterior aspect of the body

Feet → Chest → Hands

In summary, in the anatomical position of the body according to Chinese medicine, *Yang Qi* flows down from the hands through the head to the feet, and *Yin Qi* flows up from the feet through the chest to the hands.

The three levels of Yang and Yin channels: the six divisions (Liu Qi)

Early Chinese physicians realized that the interaction of Yang and Yin energy takes place in three levels of reality: heaven, earth, and the human dimension. Thus, they identified three levels of Qi channels along each aspect of the extremities. Three Yang channels flow along the posterior aspect following the lateral, intermediate, and medial surface of the extremities; and three Yin channels flow along the anterior aspect of the extremities following the medial, intermediate, and lateral surface of the extremities.

Taking as a reference the Chinese anatomical position of the body, the three levels of Yang and Yin channels are shown in Table 1.1.

Table 1.1 The three levels of Qi channels

Three Yang Channels	Three Yin Channels
Greater Yang (*Tai Yang*): Posterior lateral aspect of the extremities	Greater Yin (*Tai Yin*): Anterior medial aspect of the extremities
Lesser Yang (*Shao Yang*): Posterior intermediate aspect of the extremities	Extreme Yin (*Jue Yin*): Anterior intermediate aspect of the extremities
Yang Bright (*Yang Ming*): Posterior medial aspect of the extremities	Lesser Yin (*Shao Yin*): Anterior lateral aspect of the extremities

The hand and foot channel pairs (twelve Qi channels)

In addition, to further differentiate their connection to the twelve internal organ systems and functions of the body, the three Yang and three Yin channels are divided into those branches that go to the hands and those branches that go to the feet in the following way:

YANG CHANNELS

Hand channels: From the hands along the posterior aspect of the extremities to the head.

Foot channels: From the head along the back of the body and the posterior aspect of the legs to the feet.

YIN CHANNELS

Foot channels: From the feet along the anterior aspect of the extremities and the front of the body to the chest.

Hand channels: From the chest along the anterior aspect of the extremities to the hands.

This pattern of hand Yang channels, foot Yang channels, foot Yin channels, and hand Yin channels is repeated three times along the lateral, intermediate, and medial aspects of the extremities to make up the twelve primary Qi channels of the body. The hand and foot branches of the channels are part of the same energy layer, and run along identical anatomical aspects of the upper and lower extremities. For instance, the hand and foot greater Yang channels run along the posterior lateral aspect of the upper and lower extremities respectively.

The hand and foot branches of the channels are shown in the diagrams below.

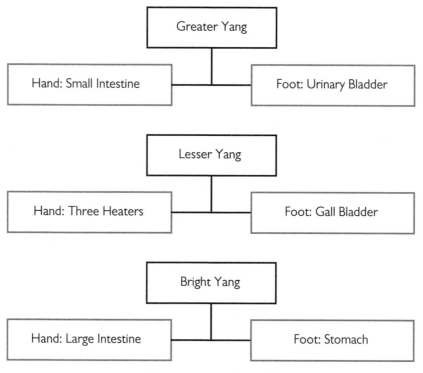

The six *Yang Qi* channels

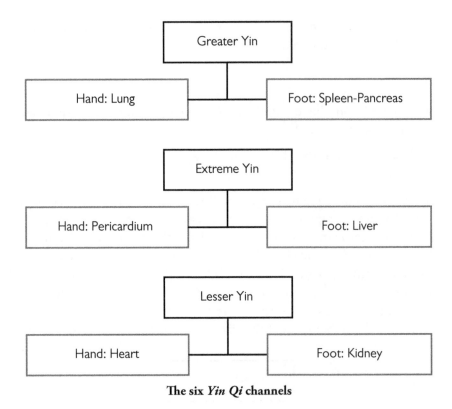

The six *Yin Qi* channels

The twelve primary Qi channels (Jing Zheng)

The twelve primary Qi channels are the main pathways for the distribution of the vital energy. The energy meridians are not just straight flat lines running along the surface of the body; rather, we should view the energy meridians as tri-dimensional fields of force that influence how particles and energy signals move through the body. They make up the energy fields in charge of signal and information transduction.

It has been suggested that information such as light, electromagnetic radiation, and subtle energy travel through the network of Qi channels, controlling the communication of biochemical messages between cells. The Qi channels work as magnetic vectors that give direction to the flow of vital energy. Also, they link the various internal organs with the external tissues, making the body an integrated whole.

Table 1.2 illustrates the twelve primary channels.

Table 1.2 The twelve primary Qi channels (*Jing Zheng*)

Six levels of Qi channels	Twelve primary Qi channels	Anatomical location
Tai Yang (Greater Yang)	Hand: Small intestines Foot: Urinary bladder	Posterior lateral aspect of the extremities
Shao Yang (Lesser Yang)	Hand: Three heaters Foot: Gall bladder	Posterior intermediate aspect of the extremities
Yang Ming (Bright Yang)	Hand: Large intestine Foot: Stomach	Posterior medial aspect of the extremities
Tai Yin (Greater Yin)	Hand: Lung Foot: Spleen	Anterior medial aspect of the extremities
Jue Yin (Extreme Yin)	Hand: Pericardium Foot: Liver	Anterior intermediate aspect of the extremities
Shao Yin (Lesser Yin)	Hand: Heart Foot: Kidney	Anterior lateral aspect of the extremities

The body clock: circadian flow of Qi

Circadian rhythms or 24-hour daily cycles are present throughout nature and influence every single living organism.

Research into chronobiology has demonstrated that cellular metabolism and the function of a variety of body systems fluctuate according to cyclic biorhythms. For instance, the production of certain hormones such as melatonin is higher at night-time and decreases during the daytime, whereas cortisol hormone decreases at night and is highest in the morning. Similarly, acid–alkaline levels, liver functions of glycogenesis and glycogenolysis, infra-orbital pressure in the eyes, cellular regeneration, and sympathetic and parasympathetic dominance, among other physiologic parameters, follow ebbs and flows according to the 24-hour cycle.

All life revolves around the cycles of nature and everything in nature is in constant motion. For instance, galaxies are constantly rotating, planets revolve around the sun as well as rotating on their own axis, and satellites orbit planets. Similarly, in the microscopic world of atoms the electrons orbit protons.

Naturally, in the human body vital energy follows a gradient flow of circulation, and thus it increases in each channel for two hours. Hence, each Qi channel and energy system of the body shows a two-hour phase of increased physiologic activity. This 24-hour cycle is known as the biological or body clock and it acts like a tidal wave with areas of increased and decreased energy, alternating between Yang and Yin phases. Thus, in 24 hours Qi makes a complete cycle through the twelve primary channels, nurturing and regulating the physiological functions of the whole body.

The body clock is illustrated on the next page.

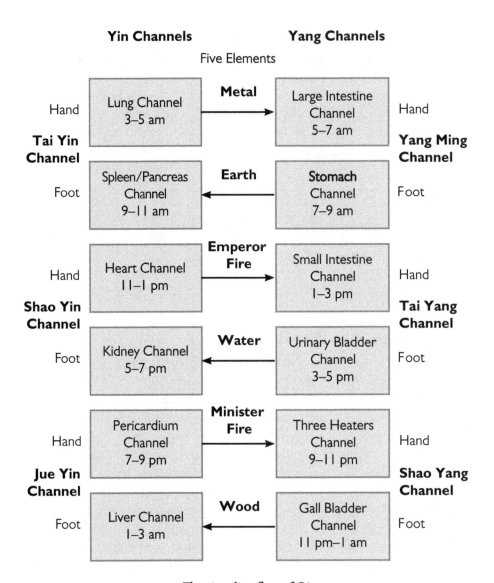

The circadian flow of Qi

Chapter 2

Principles of Practice

1. Smooth and flowing movement

Different from traditional hatha yoga poses that focus on holding a posture of the body, sequencing of body postures or intense stretching of the body, Daoist Meridian Yoga makes use of movement (*Dong*) as a means of stretching and toning the system of fascia, muscles, and connective tissue. At the same time, it alternately stretches and compresses the muscles and tendons, stimulating lymph and blood flow, thus activating the energy meridians.

The movements of Daoist Meridian Yoga are smooth and flowing in nature. They involve linking the musculoskeletal frame of the body, lengthening the connective tissue at the same time as maintaining relaxation of the muscles, cultivating Qi (energy) connectivity, and engaging the whole body in the movements.

In the system of Daoist Meridian Yoga we make use of two main levels of practice—external training and internal training:

- *External or physical training* (*Wai Gong*) refers to training and conditioning the physical body and its associated external tissues. It includes conditioning the external tissues of the body such as the muscles, joints, tendons, and external fascia.

- *Internal training* (*Nei Gong*) involves training the breathing, conditioning the internal organs and deeper tissues of the body, developing the flow of Qi, enhancing one's sensory skills, and training of the consciousness. In this way, Daoist meridian exercises require the integration of external training and internal training in order to bring about the latent potential of the body and mind.

By combining the internal and the external dimensions of training we are using the body more efficiently and are able to produce greater force. At the same time, linking the structure of the body helps to generate coherent body movement, whereas activating the flow of internal Qi improves signal transmission, and developing mind training enhances neuromuscular communication and coordination, improving overall body performance.

2. Coordinating movement and breathing

Breath is the link between the body and the mind. In the system of Chinese *Qigong* (energy exercises), breathing is seen as the power that activates the circulation of vital energy or Qi. According to *Qigong* each breathing cycle of one inhalation and one exhalation circulates vital energy approximately six body inches. Thus, deep breathing accompanied by active use of the diaphragm muscle works as a pump that helps to drive blood, fluids, and vital energy throughout the system of energy meridians.

At the same time, by focusing on coordinating the movements of the body with the breathing, we become more consciously aware of the action of the exercises upon the deeper tissues, internal organs, and energy meridians. Breathing and the flow of vital energy bring awareness to the area of the body where the breath is focused. Neglected areas of the body that we are unaware of become like "dead zones," not fully alive yet. Breathing power should be able to reach everywhere within the body without restrictions.

3. Interaction between the body and mind

There is a direct relation between the mind and vital energy. When the mind is focused and calm, vital energy is able to gather, condense, and circulate smoothly. In turn, a restless mind makes vital energy dispersed and erratic. Conversely, deep and slow breathing makes the mind calm and focused whereas short, shallow, and rapid breathing makes the mind unsettled and restless.

Wherever the mind is focused, energy follows. At the same time, the flow of vital energy brings awareness to that particular area of the body. Therefore, the movements of the body and the mind focus support each other to bring about the smooth flow of vital energy in the body.

A specific area of mind focus is given for each exercise of Daoist Meridian Yoga.

4. Stretching the body and guiding Qi

As mentioned above, *Daoyin* exercises stretch and tone the body in order to lead the flow of vital energy or Qi. In a general sense, exercise comprises three main aspects: movement, breathing, and circulation. Exercises should primarily aim at conditioning the connective tissues, improving breathing and vital lung capacity, and stimulating blood circulation. Most systems of exercise focus mainly on strengthening the physical body and cardiovascular conditioning. However, Daoist Meridian Yoga differs from regular exercise in that it not only works on conditioning the physical body, but it also enlivens the flow of internal Qi or vital energy and it seeks to strike a balance between the exterior Qi (Yang) and interior Qi (Yin) energies of the body. Focusing exclusively on physical conditioning may place undue strain on particular organs or areas of the body such as the lungs, heart, liver, and muscles, and also cause blockages of Qi in specific areas of the body.

In addition, in the practice of Daoist Meridian Yoga we emphasize the integration of the posture and movement of the body (*Xing*), the flow of internal energy (*Qi*), and the mind intent (*Yi*). Consequently, just stretching, flexing, and strengthening the body does not qualify as *Daoyin* or *Qigong* exercise. This distinct characteristic of *Daoyin* and *Qigong* exercise is expressed by a classical quote of *Qigong* practice that says: "Exercising the muscles, ligaments, and joints on the exterior of the body and exercising the deeper tissues, internal organs, Qi (vital energy), and the mind in the interior of the body."

The external motions of the body are intended to help guide the flow of internal energy. At the mature stages of practice it is the internal energy that drives the movements of the body. In effect, it is the activation and circulation of vital energy that in the long run brings the greater health benefits and well-being for the practitioner.

Thus, the ancient Chinese Qi masters sought to develop a way of exercise that would not only strengthen the exterior frame of the body, but at the same time optimize the internal functions of the body, improve health, and promote longevity.

How can we exercise the internal organs and deeper tissues of the body? Obviously, the internal organs are performing various physiologic functions according to the demands placed upon the body. However, these are mostly unconscious actions and they are not always optimal. We can bring these automatic functions to a greater level of efficiency and balance by incorporating the practices of Qi exercise through a process of inner awareness. Accordingly, in *Qigong* and Daoist Meridian Yoga the scope of internal exercise (*Nei Gong*) includes the following principles:

1. Internal stretching of the fibrous system of fascia that envelops and connects the body.

2. Opening and closing the abdominal and chest cavities in coordination with the movements of the body and the breathing.

3. Initiating the movements from the interior core of the body (*Dantian* region).

4. Engaging the deeper system of tendons and fascia while relaxing the surface muscular tissues into a deeper level of support of the body's connective tissue.

5. Conditioning of the breath along with the coordination of the breathing with the external training of the body and active use of the diaphragm muscle.

6. Gently expanding, compressing, massaging, and exercising the internal organs.

7. Activating and guiding the flow of internal Qi along the energy meridians.

8. Cultivating active relaxation of the internal organs and deeper tissues of the body.

9. Training of the consciousness and lively interaction between the body, vital energy, and the mind.

5. Maintain upper body empty and lower body full

During the Daoist Meridian Yoga exercises the upper body, including the shoulders, neck, chest, and back, is kept supple and comfortable, avoiding tension or strain. In contrast, the legs are rooted and anchored to the earth, thus facilitating grounding of the body. At the same time vital energy is gathered and circulated from the lower *Dantian* (core of the body), while the mind is kept centered and calmed.

A fundamental principle of exercise that applies to the practice of *Qigong* and *Taiji* says: "Qi is rooted in the legs, guided by the waist, circulated along the trunk, and emitted through the hands." Thus, relaxation of the upper body and grounding of the lower body are essential skills that allow vital energy to gather in the lower *Dantian*, and then circulate throughout the body.

6. Gentle and natural practice

Daoist Meridian Yoga practice should feel comfortable and natural. Do not force the position of the body, the movements, or the breath in unnatural ways. If necessary, adjust the position of the body or modify the movements to suit your present fitness level and state of health.

Chapter 3

How the Exercises Work

The five energy systems of Daoist Meridian Yoga

A fundamental notion in Chinese medicine states that most chronic diseases originate from blockages to the flow of vital energy and blood that compromise the physiological functions of the internal organs and tissues. This relation can be illustrated in a flow chart:

> Blood and energy blockages → reduced nutrients and oxygen supply → compromised organ function → build-up of toxic byproducts of metabolism → onset of chronic disease

As mentioned earlier, the system of Daoist Meridian Yoga is based on the relation between the energy pathways and the action of specific muscle groups in the body. The exercises work by rotating the joints one-by-one following a movement in a sequence, stretching and toning the tendons and lengthening two points of the body in opposite directions, thus linking the entire structure of the body. In addition, the exercises are coordinated with specific breathing techniques, mind focus, energy connectivity, and guiding Qi or vital energy to the specified area of the body.

The Daoist approach to Qi exercise includes three main aspects of practice, traditionally known as the three regulations or three adjustments (*San Tiao*):

1. *Guiding movement (Yun Dong Daoyin)*. This step refers to the positioning of the body and coordinating the movement of the body based on the requirements of each exercise.

2. *Guiding the breath (Huxi Daoyin)*. This refers to coordinating the breathing and guiding vital energy or Qi according to the specified movement and goals of the exercise.

3. *Guiding the mind (Yi Nian Daoyin)*. The final element involves making use of conscious movement and mind focus as well as coordinating the three regulations into a unified action.

Daoist Meridian Yoga exercises help in conditioning and strengthening the body, but in a way that is different from the Western view of body-building or strengthening that emphasizes developing the muscles.

With regard to physical conditioning, exercise should help accomplish three main goals: strengthening, stretching, and cardio-respiratory conditioning. Generally, body-builders tend to have shorter tendons, but larger muscle mass. That is, they gain strength to the detriment of speed and endurance. At the same time, it is estimated that muscle work accounts for much of the body's energy consumption, therefore overworking muscle tissue leads to loss of energy and fatigue. In contrast, in the system of Daoist Qi exercises we assist movement by rotating the joints so as to develop elasticity, in this way linking the musculoskeletal frame of the body. In this manner, focusing on lengthening the tendons and opening the joints helps to activate the circulation without making the muscles tight.

Maintaining body posture and generating movement is achieved by the combined action of the bones, muscles and the supporting connective tissues working together. Bones make up the dense structural framework of the body, while muscles and connective tissues serve as the flexible and contracting elements. Muscles generate force by contracting and pulling upon bones that work as levers for supporting a load or resistance acting on the body. In turn, joints function as pivot points or fulcrums for anchoring movement, assisted by the action of the connective tissues. Muscles and connective tissue have opposing and complementary roles in generating movement. Muscle action is active and contractile, while connective tissue function is supporting and elastic. Thus, as muscles stretch the tendons, fascia, and supportive tissues, the network of connective tissue, due to its elastic nature, stores tensile energy that can be used to further support subsequent movement. In this way, stretching, lengthening and toning the system of tendons and fascia increases the elasticity of the body that is the tensile energy storing capacity of connective tissues for generating greater force.

Tendons are a type of dense fibrous connective tissue that attach muscles to bones. They are tough and elastic tissues capable of absorbing and transmitting tensile forces. This mechanical property of tendons confers them with both tensile and compressive ability, allowing them to function as elastic springs. As noted above, tendons exhibit the property of elasticity that is they can stretch and then regain their contractile tone. At the same time the mechanical function of tendons and muscles is highly integrated to produce movement. This mechanical ability of resisting tensile loads and storing kinetic energy can be used as a recoil spring for generating greater power, thus allowing muscles to produce greater work and making movement more efficient.

In turn, joints are structures where bones connect to each other. They allow movement and provide mechanical support for the body. Because they make a gap between adjacent bones, blood and energy flow through the joints tends to be sluggish. Further, waste byproducts of metabolism, in particular organic acids, tend to accumulate at the joints making them stiff and achy. Thus, vital energy or Qi can easily get blocked at the joints. In the practice of *Qigong* and *Daoyin*, joints are considered as "Qi gates." When they are movable and open they allow for the free passage of vital energy and nutrients.

Biological science has developed rapidly in recent years, as has the field of exercise physiology. Several established theories and assumptions about exercise and fitness have been scrutinized and re-evaluated. It has become apparent that the traditional exercise routines of aerobics, weights, and long-distance running are not, after all, the most efficient or even safest way to achieve overall fitness and wellness.

Over the last decade or so an interesting area of research has been taking place, related to the connection between exercise and hormones. It has been found that the body releases various hormones depending on the type, intensity, and duration of exercise activity. Some of the physiological responses of the body to exercise have long been known. However, now it is possible to implement exercise programs to target a specific hormonal response of the body and accomplish precise health and wellness goals. For instance, it has been found that interval training, cross training, or high-intensity interval training (HIIT), all of which consist of repeated bouts of intense exercise followed by short rest intervals between sets, stimulate the production of testosterone, dehydroepiandrosterone (DHEA), and human growth hormone (HGH). (Testosterone is the main anabolic hormone in the body that helps build muscle mass and bone and increases sex drive, whereas the human growth hormone is secreted by the anterior pituitary gland in the brain and supports muscle growth, collagen synthesis, and joint health.) At the same time, this type of exercise improves insulin secretion and glycogen storage capacity in the muscles. In contrast, prolonged exercise stimulates the production of the thyroid hormones responsible for the metabolic rate of the body, which help to increase the burning of sugar and promote greater fatty acid utilization by the body. However, it may also activate the use of amino acids for energy production, leading to a loss of muscle mass, which in turn slows down metabolism.

In addition, aerobic exercise stimulates glucagon secretion by the pancreas, which signals the liver to release glucose into the bloodstream, and also stimulates the endorphin release that helps you to relax and feel a "natural high." However, prolonged exercise can also cause excess production of the steroid hormones cortisol and adrenalin (the so-called "stress hormones") by the adrenal glands; if this continues for an extended period of time it can lead to signs of chronic stress, including elevated blood pressure, depression, irritability, increased anxiety, chronic fatigue, insomnia, gastro-intestinal irritation, cardiovascular disease, abnormal menstrual cycles in women, decreased sex drive and fertility in men, excess fat accumulation in the abdomen, weakened immune system, and chronic inflammation. At the same time, it provokes a decrease of hormone sensitive lipase (HSL), which mobilizes free fatty acids during exercise, and diminished production of testosterone in males and estrogen in females. On the other hand, it appears that regular exercise greatly improves the sensitivity and response of the body to the action of insulin, thus decreasing insulin resistance and helping to regulate blood sugar levels. It also increases the index of leptin hormone, primarily produced by the adipose tissue of fat cells, which makes you feel satisfied and satiated after a meal and helps balance our energy metabolism.

In turn, Daoist meridian exercises and Qigong exercises have been found to have a profound regulating effect on the endocrine system and on hormonal secretions. For instance, after Qigong exercise the level of the stress hormone adrenaline decreases and at the same time the period of corticosteroid hormone exposure increases, indicating a better physiological response to stress. Qigong practice also helps improve the ratio and level of sex hormones, beta endorphins, serotonin, human growth hormone, cortisol, glucagon, and insulin, among other important parameters.

It is important to note that overtraining in any form of exercise will trigger excess cortisol release, resulting in increased protein breakdown and lowered immunity. In short, hormonal balance is essential for achieving peak levels of fitness and health.

The basic principle of Daoist Qi exercises is to guide Qi to the desired area of the body, letting Qi drive nutrients to specific tissues so that they can be strengthened and developed. At the same time the emphasis is not just on stretching the muscles, but also on toning them by pulling two opposite points of the body, while maintaining internal structural integrity, energy connectivity, and a strong rooting to the earth. Simultaneously, the exercises are coordinated with breathing techniques, mind focus, relaxation, and guiding Qi to the targeted areas. It is the synergy of these techniques that helps to open and activate the flow of vital energy along the acupuncture meridians.

For centuries, the Chinese Qi masters and internal martial artists have designed exercises and training methods to take advantage of this ability of the body to enhance human performance. Vital energy or Qi flows through a system of twelve energy pathways known as the twelve primary regular acupuncture meridians. Each energy pathway follows an external course along the surface of the body and is directly linked with an internal organ system. In addition, each energy pathway has an internal branch that travels deep within the body, and is associated with a major muscle group and specific acupuncture points or vital points located along the energy pathways. Accordingly, the system of Daoist Meridian Yoga makes use of the five systems associated with the energy pathways as described below.

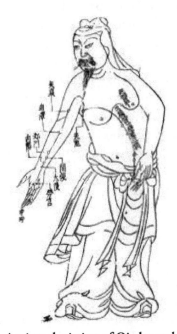

Ancient depiction of Qi channel

1. The external course of the energy pathway

Daoist Meridian Yoga is founded on the relation between the action of specific muscle groups and the energy meridians. As noted earlier, the exercises act upon and engage with the main muscle groups along the external pathway of the corresponding Qi channel.

2. The internal branches of the energy pathway

The internal branches of the Qi channels travel deep within the chest and abdominal cavities, connecting with various organ systems and tissues. The opening, closing, turning, and twisting movements of Daoist Meridian Yoga, accompanied by active use of the diaphragm and deep abdominal breathing, stimulate and provide a gentle massaging action upon the internal organs and tissues of the body.

3. The muscle groups associated with the energy pathway

As indicated, the exercises engage and act upon both the primary and secondary muscle groups connected with the energy meridians.

4. The internal organ associated with the energy pathway

The exercises stimulate important acupuncture points such as the alarm points (*Mu*) and the transport points (*Shu*) associated with the internal organs and located along the front and the back of the trunk.

5. The main vital points associated with the energy pathway

Vital energy points are located along the external course of the Qi channels along the limbs, trunk, and head. Each Daoist Meridian Yoga exercise lists the main vital points, muscle groups, Qi channels, and internal organs activated by the particular exercise.

In short, the system of Daoist Meridian Yoga comprises a comprehensive and effective method of energy balance, self-healing, and Qi fitness.

The five ways of circulating Qi in the body

According to Chinese medicine, a strong, abundant, and unrestricted flow of vital energy or Qi is the key to good health, vitality, rejuvenation, and longevity. Vigorous vital energy and smooth flow of Qi promotes optimal function of the internal organs and tissues, a strong immune system, and increased resistance to disease.

Daoist Meridian Yoga makes use of five methods to activate the flow of vital energy and blood throughout the system of energy pathways as described below.

1. Movement (*Dong*)

Naturally, physical exercise encourages faster breathing and increased blood circulation. During exercise, muscle contraction and extension stimulates blood flow to local areas, promotes tissue metabolism, and enhances the disposal of toxic byproducts of metabolism. Likewise, it is well-known that muscular movement is the primary means to stimulate lymph flow in the body. Unlike the vascular system of blood vessels and capillaries, the lymphatic system doesn't have the pumping power of the heart, but relies on muscle action to keep it moving. It is the alternating contraction and relaxation of the muscular tissue that acts as a pumping mechanism for the system of lymph vessels.

Furthermore, lymphatic flow and Qi circulation mutually influence one another. Lymph is the main extracellular fluid circulating in the space outside and around the cells. At the same time, Qi or vital energy flows through the system of fascia and connective tissue that surrounds the cells and organs of the body. Thus, physical exercise drives proper circulation of lymphatic fluids, which in turn helps to promote the flow of Qi in the body.

It is well-documented that most forms of exercise provide several fitness benefits. The various approaches to exercise bring their own advantages depending on the individual's specific motivations and goals. The main difference between them is that external exercise systems emphasize the use of localized muscular force and body power, while internal exercise systems utilize a coherent whole-body motion, the elastic spring force of the body's connective tissue network, the mind leading Qi or vital energy, and Qi fueling the movements of the body. Another important aspect of the Daoist approach to exercise for overall health and wellness involves building up and strengthening the supply of post-natal energy—the Qi acquired after birth (*Zhen Qi*) from breath, nutrients, and movement—so that we don't have to tap into and deplete our capital of original Qi (*Yuan Qi*). For instance, moderate exercise such as brisk walking, light weights, and resistance exercise, and some forms of interval training help to improve a great number of markers of fitness, including building and maintaining muscle mass, strengthening the heart, improving cardio-respiratory function, and stimulating fat metabolism. However, not every kind of exercise can bring about these desired benefits. In effect, exercises that involve excessive and sustained muscular force or repetitive mechanical movement favoring specific muscle groups actually create muscle tightness and fatigue. Similarly, extreme aerobic exercise that incurs a deficit of oxygen supply increases lactic acid build-up in the tissues, which makes your muscles tight and thus results in restricted Qi and blood flow.

Statistical studies have shown that, although professional endurance athletes are fitter and have much better cardiovascular health, on average they live shorter lives than the general population. How is that possible? It is because excessive aerobic exercise as well as exaggerated body-building places a significant strain on specific systems of the body such as the heart, lungs, liver, muscles, and joints. In addition, exercising too intensely may weaken the immune system, disrupt hormonal balance, increase the production of damaging free radicals, impair cellular integrity, and compromise other vital functions of the body. Over time, this strain on the body consumes and depletes our vital energy reserves of *Yuan Qi* (original Qi).

Other important considerations when exercising include balancing the external training of the connective tissues with the conditioning of the internal organs and vital energy, exercising opposing muscle groups as well as the upper and lower body, improving both muscle strength and muscle flexibility. Excessive focus on muscle building and strength causes shortening, tightness, and contraction of the tissues. On the other hand, too much emphasis on stretching and flexibility causes the muscles to lose proper tone, making them weaker. Again, the answer lies in the proper balance between muscle strength and flexibility, which provides the drive for optimal blood and Qi circulation.

In Eastern medicine the view of health goes well beyond muscles and cardiovascular fitness. In both traditions of yoga and *Qigong* the definition of true health encompasses a much broader scope that includes the following criteria:

1. Optimal physiological function of the internal organ systems of the body.

2. Proper digestive function, assimilation of nutrients, and disposal of waste.

3. Strong immune system and active resistance to disease.

4. Balance of the five elements and their related functions and tissues.

5. Sustained energy level and vitality.

6. Fine functioning of the five senses: vision, hearing, smell, taste, and touch.

7. Balanced expression of emotions.

8. A peaceful state of mind and inner contentment.

2. Breathing (*Tiao Xi*)

Breathing is our most vital function of survival. It goes on automatically at all times about ten to 14 times per minute without our conscious awareness. The automatic nature of breathing is essential to our survival as every cell in the body needs a constant oxygen supply. In particular, brain cells are especially sensitive to lack of oxygen and if deprived for even a few minutes they will die, not to be replaced.

In Chinese medicine the lungs are referred to as "the masters of Qi." Breathing brings in the clear Qi (*Qing Qi*) and oxygen from air which diffuses from the bronchi into the capillaries of the blood. Oxygen is taken up by the blood and goes to the heart, from where it is delivered through the vascular system carrying vital energy and nutrients to every single cell in the body. Consequently, proper and efficient breathing is essential for oxygenating the tissues, activating the physiological functions of the body, stimulating metabolism, and driving the movement of Qi, blood, and body fluids. As mentioned earlier, each breath moves vital energy by about six body inches. Thus, in Daoist Meridian Yoga breath is used as a tool to control and guide the movement of vital energy. The exercises and movements of the body should be combined with the breathing in order to achieve optimal results.

3. Mind focus (*Yi*)

In the method of Chinese internal exercise the relationship between Qi and the mind is expressed by a principle of guiding energy that says: "The mind leads the Qi and Qi is the vehicle for the mind." Accordingly, where the mind is focused the Qi follows.

Initially, it is not easy to direct the movement of Qi with the mind alone. Strengthening vital energy and developing the sensation of Qi inside the body facilitates connecting the mind with the flow of internal energy. This is known as *Qigang* or the experience and sensation of Qi. Once the feeling of Qi is strong, the mind will be naturally attracted to the flow of internal Qi.

There are various methods used in *Qigong* for focusing or concentrating the mind. In the system of Daoist Meridian Yoga we focus on specific vital points and areas of the body to direct the flow of Qi and activate the energy meridians.

4. Relaxation (*Song*)

Relaxation stimulates the vagus or parasympathetic nervous system, promoting dilation of blood vessels, increased microcirculation to the extremities, and opening of the Qi channels.

The Chinese term for relaxation is *Song*. It means to loosen up and let go of excessive muscular tension. It also means extending, expanding, and opening, as in extending the body and opening the flow of Qi.

Therefore, in Daoist Meridian Yoga relaxation is not totally slack or limp. Within relaxation there must be a feeling of extension, inner expansion, flow of Qi, and mind focus. It is an "active relaxation" in which, through a process of inner awareness and receptivity, the mind controls the relaxation response of the nervous system and the physical body. At the same time, the skill of relaxation is not just limited to the external tissues or muscles, but should be extended to the deeper tissues of the body, internal organs, nervous system, and the mind. In particular, the relaxation of the mind is essential. Tension in the mind creates nervous tension, which in turn triggers physical tension. Therefore, relaxation of the mind is of foremost importance for achieving overall relaxation.

5. Practicing with the *Dantian* as the center (*Dantian Wei Hexin*)

The *Dantian* is the root of Qi or vital energy in the human body as well as the anatomical center of gravity of the body.

Dantian is a term used in *Qigong*, meaning "field of elixir." The first character, *Dan*, represents a cauldron or pot in which a pill, medicine, or elixir is prepared.

In this context, the "elixir" refers to the original Qi or vital energy inside the body. The second character, *Tian*, shows the image of a field or area for the growing of crops. It actually indicates the area of the lower abdomen at the core of the body. Thus, the *Dantian* is the area where the original Qi of the body can be harnessed, cultivated, and nurtured.

Practicing with the *Dantian* as the center means that the various movements of Daoist Meridian Yoga should be connected with the movement of the *Dantian* region and they must follow the turning, rotating, opening, closing, and spiraling motions of the *Dantian*. In addition, during the performance of the exercises vital energy is gathered and issued from the *Dantian* center.

All the energy channels originate from the *Dantian*. In the yoga tradition this region is known as the *Kanda* and it is the root of all the *nadis* or currents of *prana* (life force). Thus, the *Dantian* is regarded as the nucleus of vital energy and the main storehouse of Qi for the whole body.

Daoist Meridian Yoga exercises differ from regular exercise in that the limbs do not move independently of the *Dantian*, and every movement of the body is connected to the *Dantian* center.

Guide to practicing the exercises

Daoist Meridian Yoga exercises are organized into three groups of four related energy pathways, following the 24-hour cycle of Qi flow along the twelve energy meridians. Two exercises are designed for each energy pathway. Thus, the whole set of Daoist Meridian Yoga is comprised of 24 exercises.

The exercises of Daoist Meridian Yoga can be practiced in four ways according to the specific needs, interests, and goals of the individual:

1. As single exercise to stimulate the flow of Qi along a specific energy pathway and related internal organ.

2. As a pair of exercises to activate and balance coupled Yang and Yin energy pathways and their related organs within the same element according to the five elements of Chinese medicine:

   1. *Metal element*: Lung and large intestine Qi channels.

   2. *Earth element*: Stomach and spleen Qi channels.

   3. *Fire element*: Heart and small intestine Qi channels.

   4. *Water element*: Urinary bladder and kidney Qi channels.

   5. *Minister fire element*: Pericardium and three heaters Qi channels.

   6. *Wood element*: Gall bladder and liver Qi channels.

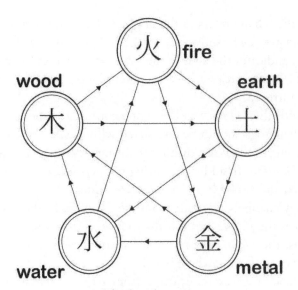

The five elements

3. As a group of four related energy pathways and organ systems following the daily cycle of Qi flow in the body:

    • *First group*: Lung, large intestine, stomach, and spleen Qi channels.

    • *Second group*: Heart, small intestine, urinary bladder, and kidney Qi channels.

    • *Third group*: Pericardium, three heaters, gall bladder, and liver Qi channels.

4. As a set of 24 exercises for a complete meridian workout, overall Qi balancing, and self-healing practice.

Part II

STEP-BY-STEP DESCRIPTION OF THE EXERCISES

The following chapters give a step-by-step description of the exercises for each energy meridian.

Note: The descriptions of the Qi channels are made taking as a reference the standard Western anatomical position of the body. In this position the body is standing with the arms down by the sides and palms facing the front.

The muscles set in bold type indicate either the primary muscle groups activated by the exercise or muscle groups that are directly associated with the pathway of the corresponding Qi channel.

Introduction to the Exercises

Below there is a description of the opening exercise and a list of the abbreviations used in the diagrams showing the twelve Qi channels. The opening exercise should be performed three times before starting the practice of the exercises, then once at the end of each individual exercise, and finally three times at the end of the exercises.

Abbreviations for the twelve regular Qi channels

L: Lung

LI: Large intestine

ST: Stomach

SP: Spleen

HT: Heart

SI: Small intestine

BL: Urinary bladder

Kd: Kidney

P: Pericardium

TH: Three heaters

GB: Gall bladder

LV: Liver

CIRCULATING THE BREATH

Starting position

Stand with the feet shoulder-width apart and the hands by the sides.

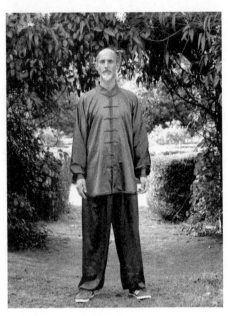

Description of the exercise

I Slowly raise the hands with palms up along the sides of the body to the top of the head as you breathe in.

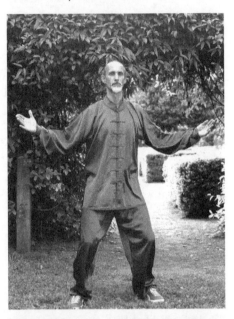

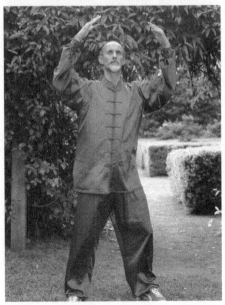

CIRCULATING THE BREATH

2 Turn the palms down and lower the hands along the front of the body to the lower abdomen area (lower *Dantian*). At the same time bend the knees, lowering the body as you breathe out.

3 Repeat the movement three times.

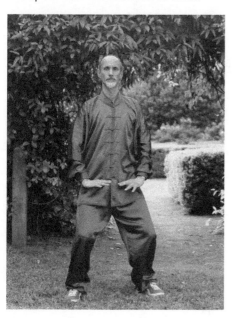

Observations

‣ When raising the hands and breathing in, focus on circulating Qi up the governing vessel (*Du Mai*), which runs up along the posterior midline of the body. When lowering the hands and breathing out, focus on circulating Qi down the conception vessel (*Ren Mai*), which runs down along the posterior midline of the body.

‣ When the hands reach the top of the head, focus on absorbing Qi from heaven into the *Bai Hui* point located on the vertex of the head.

‣ Raise and lower the body along with the movement of the hands.

‣ Keep the shoulders lowered and the hands relaxed.

Chapter 4

Daoist Yoga Exercises for the Lung Energy Meridian

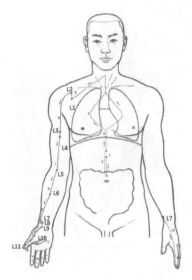

Lung Qi channel

Pathway of the Qi channel

The lung channel starts from the area of the stomach in the middle abdomen and descends to connect with the large intestines. It then curves up and ascends along the abdomen, crosses through the diaphragm, enters the lungs, and comes out to the surface of the body at the lateral corner of the chest. The channel continues traveling down the anterior lateral aspect of the upper arm, elbow, and lower arm. It then reaches the radial (thumb) side of the wrist, follows along the base of the thumb, and ends at the lateral side of the thumb. This channel has eleven vital points.

Internal branches

1. From the stomach area in the middle abdomen a branch comes down to the large intestine and then goes up through the diaphragm into the chest, throat, and lungs.

2. From the bone just above the wrist (styloid process) a branch runs across the dorsum of the hand to the lateral side of the index finger.

Main signs of imbalance

Signs of excess (Fullness of Qi)

Fullness and oppression in the chest, cough with productive phlegm and mucus, congestion of the chest, coarse breathing, difficult breathing (dyspnea), asthma with phlegm in the chest, nasal congestion, fever and chills, common cold, sore throat, nosebleed, heat in the palm, pain in the chest, shoulder, upper back and armpit, lumps and pain in the ribs, and pain along the course of the channel.

Signs of weakness (Emptiness of Qi)

Weak and shallow breathing, shortness of breath, asthma with weakness of the lungs, wheezing, weak or dry cough, weak voice, spontaneous sweating, dry throat, frequent colds with poor resistance to disease, some types of allergic reactions, sensitivity and dislike of cold, and frequent yawning.

Main areas covered

Stomach, large intestine, diaphragm, lungs, throat, chest, anterior lateral aspect of upper arm, elbow and forearm, radial side of wrist, and thumb.

PICK FRUITS

Main vital points

Conception Vessel 6 (sea of Qi) located two fingers below the navel, Conception Vessel 12 (middle stomach) four inches above the navel, Conception Vessel 15 (below sternum) just below the chest bone, Conception Vessel 17 (middle of the breasts) on the center of the chest, Lung 1 (central mansion) on the lateral corner of the chest, Lung 10 (fish belly) at the midpoint of the base of the thumb, Lung 11 (lesser *Shang*) at the lateral side of the thumb.

Main muscle groups

Anterior deltoid (anterior aspect of shoulder between lateral collar bone and upper arm), **pectoralis major** (chest region from chest bone and medial collar bone to upper arm), **teres major** (from inferior angle of shoulder blade to medial aspect of upper arm), latissimus dorsi (from crest of hip bone, sacrum, and lower thoracic vertebrae across middle and lower back to posterior aspect of upper arm), anterior serratus (chest wall between outer surface of upper 8 ribs and anterior aspect of shoulder blade), **diaphragm** (between thoracic and abdominal cavities horizontally around lower back, ribs and chest bone).

Secondary muscle groups

Subscapularis (anterior aspect of shoulder blade), external oblique (lateral aspect of abdomen from lower 8 ribs to abdomen and hip bone), internal oblique (lateral aspect of abdomen from anterior hip bone to lower 4 ribs and abdomen), **intercostals** (between ribs), erector spinae (along back between vertebrae, posterior ribs, and occipital bone), transversospinalis (along back between transverse processes and spinous processes of vertebrae).

Starting position

Stand with the feet together and hands by the sides.

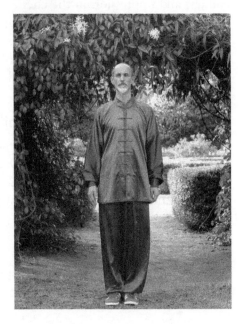

PICK FRUITS

Description of the exercise

1 Turn the body from the waist to the left side reaching up with the right arm and describing an inward rotation as if reaching to grab a fruit from a tree branch.

2 Repeat the movement with the left arm, this time turning the body to the right side and reaching up with the left arm. At the same time rotate the right arm down and out to the side of the right shoulder.

3 Alternate the movement of the arms to the left and right sides for several times.

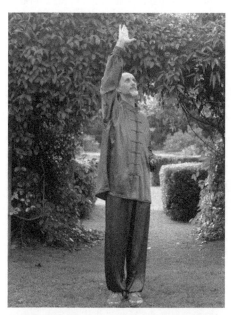

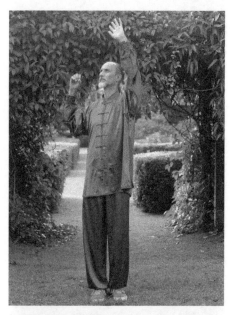

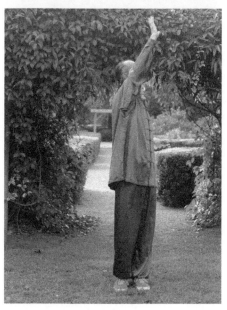

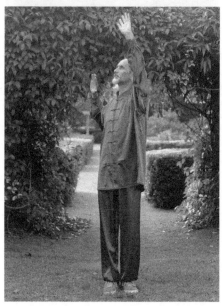

PICK FRUITS

4 End by stepping out with the left foot and lowering the hands down the front of the body to the lower *Dantian*.

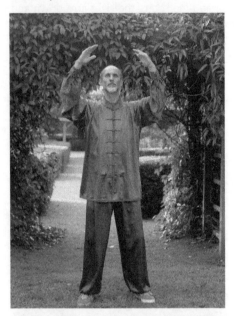

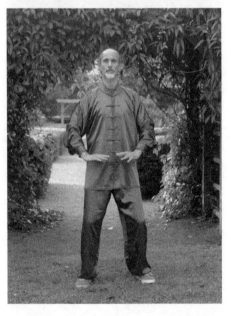

Observations

‣ Turn the body from the waist and not just from the shoulders.

‣ Try opening the ribs on the same side of the arm that is reaching up and keeping the shoulders lowered throughout.

‣ Focus the mind on the lung Qi channel extending from the chest up the arm to the thumb.

Precautions and contraindications

This exercise can be contraindicated in cases of painful conditions of the shoulder.

Breathing method

Breathe in when reaching up with one hand and breathe out when reaching up with the opposite hand. Breathe out when lowering the hands down the front of the body.

PICK FRUITS

Flow of Qi

When reaching up with the arm, vital energy flows from the lower abdomen up the middle abdomen to the chest, and up the arm along the lung Qi channel to the thumb and first finger of the hand. When lowering the hands in front of the body, Qi flows back to the *Dantian* center.

Mind focus

Focus on reaching up with the arm, turning the body from the waist, and connecting the movement of the body from the feet up the trunk to the arms and hands.

Main Qi channel

Lung.

Secondary Qi channels

Stomach, large intestine, conception vessel (*Ren Mai*).

Main benefits

- Releases tension of the diaphragm and stimulates breathing.

- Stretches the ribs and opens up the rib cage.

- Loosens up the joints of the whole body and awakens the spine.

- Helps to awaken the Qi or vital energy.

- Works out the chest, shoulders and arms.

- Stimulates the flow of Qi along the lung channel.

- Improves bowel function.

PARTING CLOUDS WITH THE HANDS

Main vital points

Lung 1 (central mansion) on the corner of the chest, Large Intestine 15 (shoulder bone) on the anterior lateral aspect of the shoulder, Pericardium 8 (labored palace) on the center of the palm between the second and third metacarpal bones, Lung 11 (lesser *Shang*) at the lateral side of the thumb, Large Intestine 11 (pool at the bend) at the end of the lateral elbow crease when the elbow is bent.

Main muscle groups

Biceps brachii (anterior aspect of upper arm), **posterior deltoid** (posterior aspect of shoulder between shoulder blade and upper arm), **infraspinatus** (shoulder blade region), teres minor (lateral inferior aspect of shoulder blade), supraspinatus (superior aspect of shoulder blade), middle trapezius (upper back area from thoracic vertebrae to spine of shoulder blade), **rhomboids** (shoulder blade area from thoracic vertebrae to medial border of shoulder blade), **coracobrachialis** (anterior medial aspect of upper arm), pectoralis major (chest region from chest bone and medial collar bone to upper arm).

Secondary muscle groups

Supinator (lateral superior aspect of forearm), pronator teres (anterior aspect of forearm across from medial elbow to middle of lateral radius bone), pronator quadratus (horizontally across proximal aspect of wrist), gluteus maximus (buttock area from hip bone to lateral aspect of thigh).

Starting position

Standing with the feet parallel and shoulder-width apart, turn the right foot out 45 degrees, and step out to the front with the left foot into a forward bow stance. Keep the weight on the rear leg and the feet shoulder-width apart.

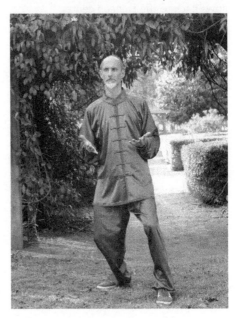

PARTING CLOUDS WITH THE HANDS

Description of the exercise

1 Place the hands by the sides of the ribs with the palms facing up.

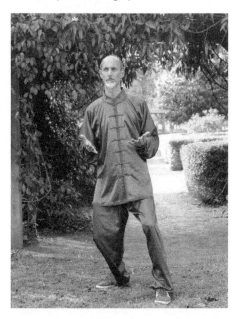

2 Extend the arms to the front with the palms up while hollowing the chest. At the same time shift the weight into the front leg, breathing out.

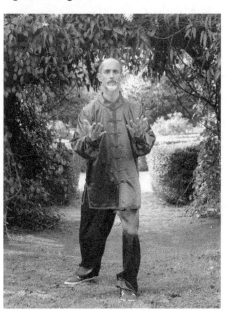

3 Rotate the hands out, extending the arms to the sides and shifting the weight to the rear leg. At the same time open the chest, breathing in.

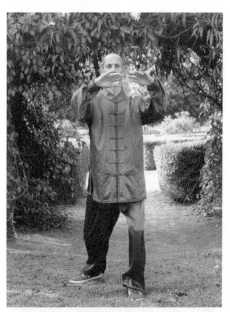

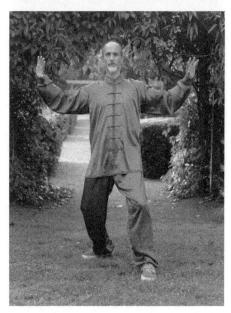

PARTING CLOUDS WITH THE HANDS

4 Rotate the hands down and inward toward the ribs turning the palms up as you breathe out.

5 Repeat the movement several times.

6 With the weight on the rear leg and arms extended out to the sides, turn the palms to face the front and move the arms forward shifting the weight to the front leg.

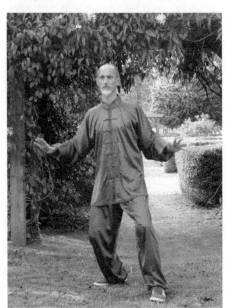

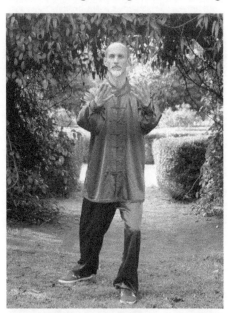

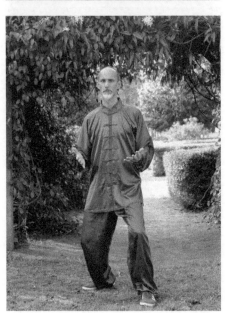

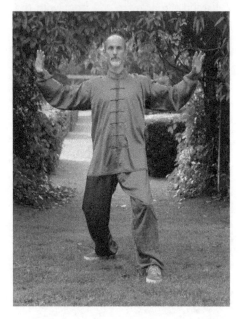

PARTING CLOUDS WITH THE HANDS

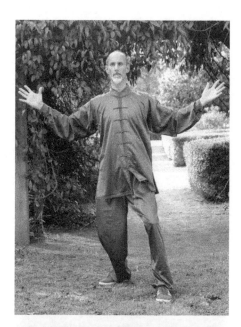

7 Bend the elbows, bringing the hands to the chest with palms facing the body. At the same time shift the weight to the rear leg, breathing in.

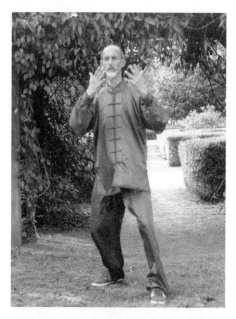

8 Rotate the palms out and push the hands to the front, shifting weight to the front leg and breathing out.

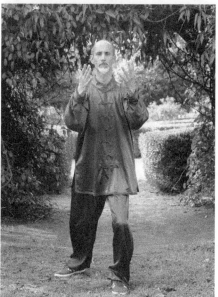

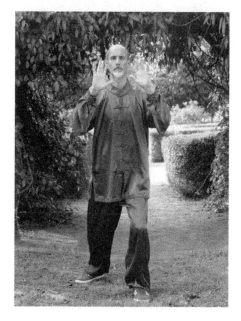

PARTING CLOUDS WITH THE HANDS

9 Rotate the hands out, extending the arms to the sides and shifting the weight to the rear leg, breathing in.

10 Repeat steps 6 through 9 two more times.

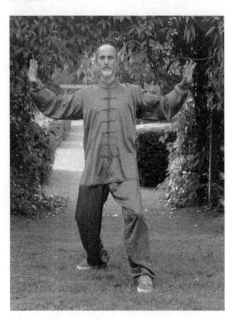

11 End by stepping back with the left foot and bringing the hands down to the lower *Dantian*.

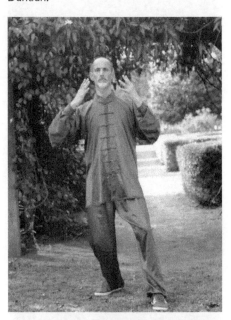

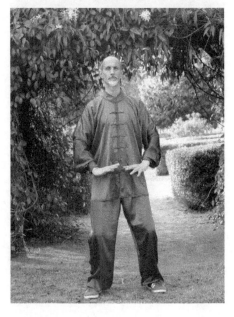

PARTING CLOUDS WITH THE HANDS

12 Step into a forward bow stance with the right foot in front and repeat the exercise on the right side.

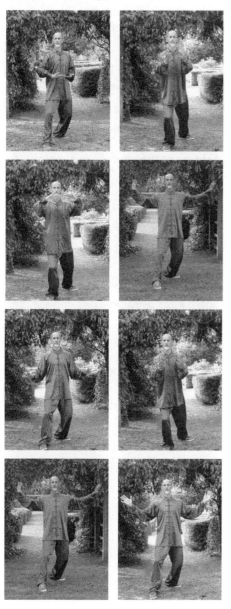

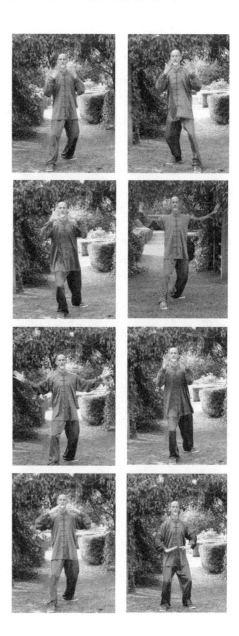

PARTING CLOUDS WITH THE HANDS

Observations

‣ Focus on opening and closing the chest in coordination with the movement of the arms and the breathing.

‣ When extending the hands to the sides, parting the clouds and opening the chest, imagine breathing in Qi of bright white color into the lungs.

‣ Keep the shoulders lowered and wrists relaxed throughout the exercise.

Breathing method

Breathe in when extending the hands out at the sides, when bending the arms bringing the hands to the chest, and when opening the chest. Breathe out when pushing the hands out to the front and when closing the chest.

Flow of Qi

Qi flows from the lower *Dantian* to the chest and out from the arms along the lung and large intestine Qi channels to the hands.

Mind focus

Focus on coordinating the movements of the body with the breathing, opening and closing the chest, and the sensation of parting the clouds with the hands.

Main Qi channel

Lung.

Secondary Qi channels

Large intestine, pericardium.

Main benefits

‣ Opens up the chest and stimulates breathing.

‣ Expands the rib cage, increasing breathing capacity.

‣ Helps to loosen up the upper back, chest, and diaphragm.

‣ Stimulates deep breathing through the abdomen.

‣ Increases flexibility of the shoulders.

Chapter 5

Daoist Yoga Exercises for the Large Intestine Energy Meridian

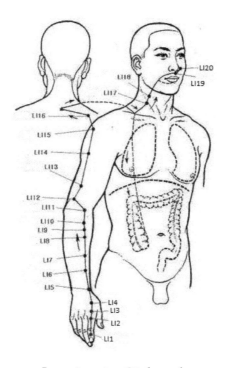

Large intestine Qi channel

Pathway of the Qi channel

The large intestine channel starts from the lateral side of the index finger, runs up the radial side of the first finger, follows over the dorsum of the hand between the first and second metacarpal bones, and reaches the lateral aspect of the wrist. It then travels up the posterior lateral aspect of the forearm, the lateral aspect of the elbow crease, and up the posterior lateral aspect of the upper arm to the shoulder joint. The channel continues over the shoulder, moves up the anterior aspect of the neck to the face, and crosses the area under the nose ending at the opposite side of the nose. This channel has 20 vital points.

Internal branches

1. From the shoulder a branch travels over the collar bone connecting to the lungs, moves the diaphragm, and enters the large intestine.

2. From the depression above the collar bone a branch travels up the neck, turns to the cheek, enters the lower gums, and skirts around the lips.

3. A branch comes out from the large intestine and travels down to the lower leg to a point six inches below the knee (Stomach 37).

4. From the side of the nose a branch connects to the inner corner of the eye.

Main signs of imbalance

Signs of excess (Fullness of Qi)

Lower abdominal pain and distension, gas, rumbling of the intestines (borborygmus), constipation, dysentery, colitis, inflammatory bowel disease, ulcerative colitis, mucus in the stool, gastro-enteritis, excretion of thick, slimy, and yellow matter, fever, sore or swollen throat, nosebleed, toothache, pain and redness of the eyes, pain and swelling of the neck, redness and pain of the fingers, frontal headache, tooth decay, shoulder joint pain, elbow pain, difficulty lifting the arm, difficulty turning the neck to the left or right, paralysis of the upper limbs, and sensations of pain, spasm, stiffness, heat, or swelling along the course of the Qi channel.

Signs of weakness (Emptiness of Qi)

Thin stool or diarrhea, rumbling of the intestines (borborygmus), sensation of coldness in the abdomen, sensitivity of teeth to cold, lack of tone or weakness of the muscles along the course of the Qi channel, and sensation of coldness along the channel.

Main areas covered

Index finger, back of the hand between thumb and first finger, radial side of wrist, posterior lateral aspect of forearm, lateral aspect of elbow, posterior lateral aspect of upper arm, lateral aspect of shoulder, shoulder joint, anterior lateral aspect of neck, lower gums, face, nose, lung, diaphragm, large intestine, and lateral aspect of lower leg.

WHITE CRANE SPREADS ITS WINGS

Main vital points

Large Intestine 15 (shoulder bone) lateral anterior to the shoulder joint, Large Intestine 11 (pool at the bend) at the lateral crease of the elbow, Large Intestine 4 (joined valleys) on the dorsum of the hand between the thumb and the first finger, Conception Vessel 6 (sea of Qi) two fingers below the navel, Conception Vessel 17 (middle of the breasts) at the center of the chest, Urinary Bladder 25 (large intestine transport) one and a half inches from the fourth lumbar vertebra, Stomach 25 (celestial pivot) two inches lateral to the navel, Stomach 37 (upper great hollow) six inches below the lateral inferior end of the kneecap.

Main muscle groups

Middle deltoid (lateral aspect of shoulder on upper arm), supraspinatus (superior aspect of shoulder blade), triceps (posterior aspect of upper arm between upper arm and elbow), latissimus dorsi (from crest of hip bone, sacrum, and lower thoracic vertebrae across middle and lower back to posterior aspect of upper arm), **infraspinatus** (shoulder blade region), teres minor (lateral inferior aspect of shoulder blade), **posterior deltoid** (posterior aspect of shoulder between shoulder blade and upper arm), **rectus abdominis** (anterior aspect of abdomen between pubic bone and lower end of chest bone), **internal oblique** (lateral aspect of abdomen from anterior hip bone to lower 4 ribs and abdomen), **rhomboids** (shoulder blade area from thoracic vertebrae to medial border of shoulder blade), middle trapezius (upper back area from thoracic vertebrae to spine of shoulder blade), **hamstrings** (posterior aspect of thigh between sitting bone and posterior knee), popliteus (posterior aspect of knee).

Secondary muscle groups

Pectoralis major (chest region from chest bone and medial collar bone to upper arm), pronator quadratus (horizontally across anterior inferior aspect of forearm and proximal to wrist), pronator teres (anterior aspect of forearm across from medial elbow to middle of lateral radius bone), brachialis (anterior inferior aspect of upper arm between upper arm bone and ulna bone), upper trapezius (neck and shoulder region between neck vertebrae and lateral aspect of collar bone), teres major (from inferior angle of shoulder blade to medial aspect of upper arm), rectus femoris (anterior aspect of thigh between pelvis and kneecap), tibialis anterior (anterior aspect of lower leg on shin bone).

Starting position

Stand with the feet together and hands by the sides.

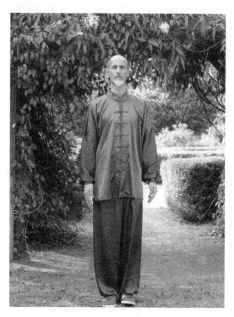

WHITE CRANE SPREADS ITS WINGS

Description of the exercise

1 Raise the hands up the sides of the body to shoulder level with the wrists loose while breathing in.

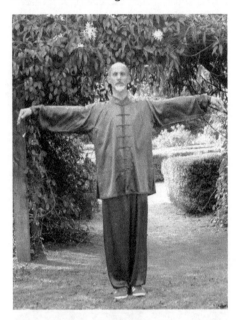

2 Extend the hands to the front at chest level, bringing the palms together.

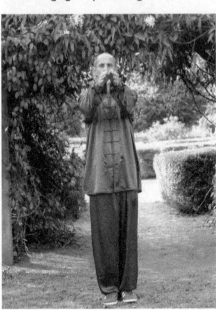

3 Turn the palms out, bringing the back of the hands together.

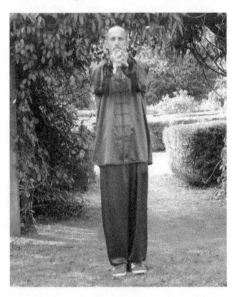

4 Move the hands down to the lower abdomen. Then bring the hands in and up the midline of the body to chest level while breathing in. In a continuous manner move the hands out to the front and down to the abdomen with the back of the hands held together while breathing out.

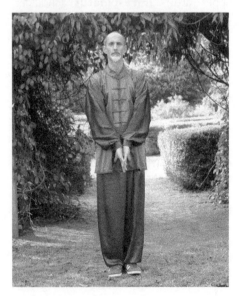

WHITE CRANE SPREADS ITS WINGS

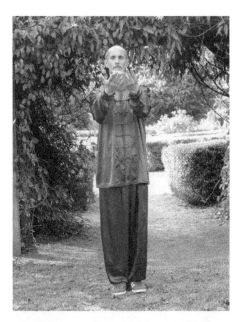

5 Bring the hands back behind the body, rolling the shoulders back and crossing the right thumb over the left thumb. At the same time lean the body back while breathing in.

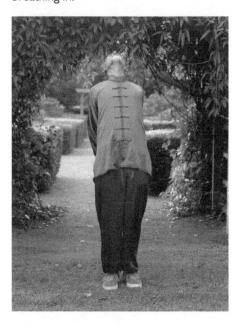

6 Bend the body down from the hips, extending the arms up behind the back and breathing out. Hold this position while taking three deep breaths from the abdomen.

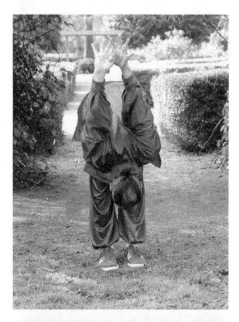

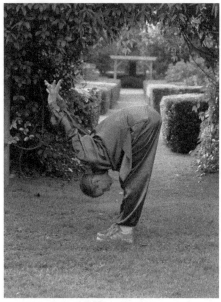

WHITE CRANE SPREADS ITS WINGS

7 Squat down or bend the knees, interlocking the ends of the fingers of both hands.

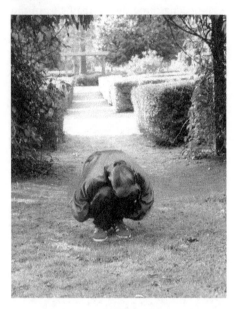

8 Bring the hands under the buttocks with fingers held together, stretching the shoulder blade area while breathing out.

9 Slowly straighten up the body, bringing the hands out to the front and up to chest level while breathing in.

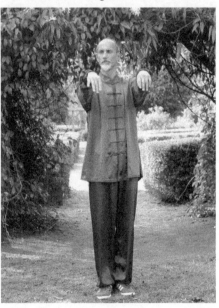

10 Move the hands down to the lower abdomen. Then bring the back of the hands together and move the hands up the midline of the body to chest level as you breathe in. In a continuous motion bring the hands out and down the front of the body and then back behind the body rolling the shoulders back, this time crossing the left thumb over the right thumb.

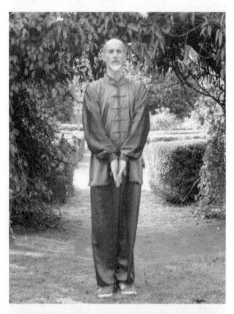

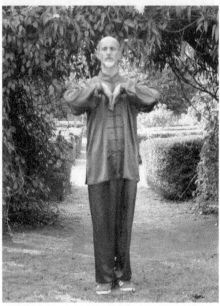

WHITE CRANE SPREADS ITS WINGS

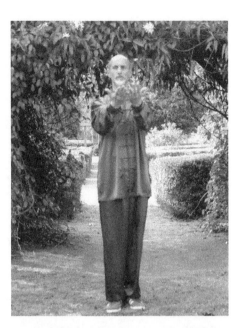

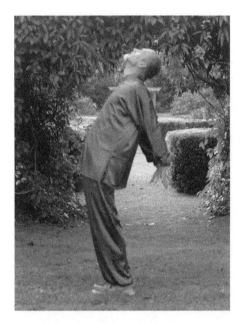

11 Lean the body back while breathing in.

12 Bend the body from the hips, repeating the exercise as before.

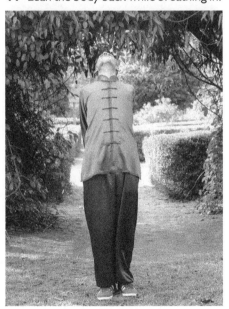

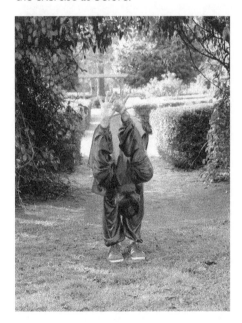

WHITE CRANE SPREADS ITS WINGS

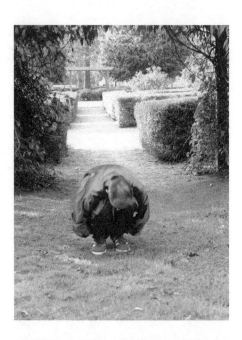

Observations

‣ The mind focus should be placed on bending from the hips and not the back, folding at the lower abdomen, and stretching the shoulder blade area.

‣ Keep the shoulders lowered throughout the exercise.

‣ Crossing the thumbs and stretching the arms back activates the large intestine Qi channel.

‣ Bending the body at the hips compresses and massages Stomach 25, the alarm point for the large intestine located two inches lateral to the navel. This action also stretches Urinary Bladder 25, the transport point of the large intestine located on the lower back.

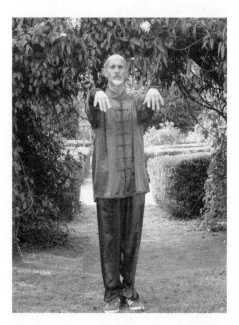

13 End by bringing the hands down the front of the body to the lower *Dantian*.

WHITE CRANE SPREADS ITS WINGS

- Bending at the hips stretches the hamstrings and lumbar muscles, which are two of the main muscle groups associated with the large intestine.

- Squatting down relaxes the rectum and the last segment of the large intestine.

Precautions and contraindications
This exercise is contraindicated in cases of slipped disc, serious lower back conditions, sciatica, high blood pressure, vertigo, heart disease, stroke, and painful conditions of the shoulder joint.

Breathing method
Breathe in when raising the hands, when leaning the body back, and when squatting down. Breathe out when lowering the hands, when bending the body down, and when moving the hands under the buttocks.

Flow of Qi
Qi flows up the trunk to the chest and up the arm along the large intestine Qi channel. When bending the body and squatting, Qi flows down the lower abdomen and the large intestine.

Mind focus
Focus on coordinating the movements of the body with the breathing, and the flow of Qi up the chest and arms and down the abdomen.

Main Qi channel
Large intestine.

Secondary Qi channels
Three heaters, conception vessel (*Ren Mai*), urinary bladder.

Main benefits

- Stimulates peristalsis and bowel motility.

- Provides a massaging action on the intestinal tract and digestive organs by stretching and compressing the abdomen.

- Helps to release spasms of the rectum, alleviating constipation.

- Stretches the shoulder muscles along the path of the large intestine Qi channel.

- Loosens up the shoulder blade area, unblocking nervous and emotional tension.

- Stretches the lower back and the hamstring muscle groups, which are two reflex areas associated with the large intestine Qi channel.

GOLDEN ROOSTER STANDS ON ONE LEG

Main vital points

Large Intestine 15 (shoulder bone) on the anterior lateral aspect of the shoulder joint, Stomach 25 (celestial pivot) two inches lateral from the navel, Urinary Bladder 25 (large intestine transport) two fingers lateral to the fourth lumbar vertebra, Stomach 37 (upper great hollow) six inches below the lateral inferior border of the kneecap, Kidney 1 (gushing spring) on the bottom of the feet.

Main muscle groups

Iliopsoas (core muscles between lumbar vertebrae and head of thigh bone), rectus femoris (anterior aspect of thigh between pelvis and kneecap), pectineus (upper inner aspect of thigh between pubic bone and thigh bone), **tensor fascia latae** (lateral aspect of thigh between crest of hip bone and lateral aspect of knee), **quadratus lumborum** (lower back area between posterior hip bone and lumbar vertebrae), gluteus maximus (buttock area from hip bone to lateral aspect of thigh), rectus abdominis (anterior aspect of abdomen between pubic bone and lower end of chest bone).

Secondary muscle groups

Biceps brachii (anterior aspect of upper arm), brachialis (anterior inferior aspect of upper arm between upper arm bone and ulna bone), sartorius (anterior aspect of thigh between anterior superior hip bone and medial aspect of knee), adductor longus and adductor brevis (upper inner thigh between pubic bone and thigh bone).

Starting position

Stand with the feet together and hands by the sides.

Description of the exercise

1 Raise the hands up the sides of the body to shoulder level with the thumb and first finger held together making a ring. At the same time turn the head to the right side.

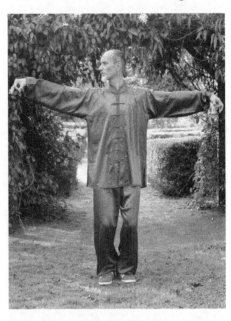

2 Step back with the right foot, shift the weight to the right leg, and bring the hands down to the lower *Dantian*.

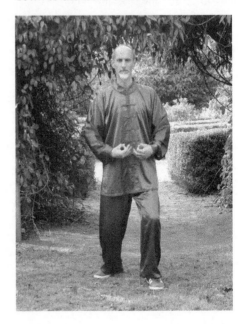

GOLDEN ROOSTER STANDS ON ONE LEG

3 Raise the hands up the sides of the body with the thumb and first finger held together. At the same time turn the head to the left side.

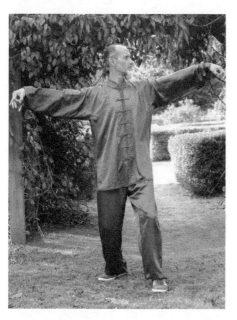

4 Lower the hands down the sides and rotate the hands toward the back facing the body.

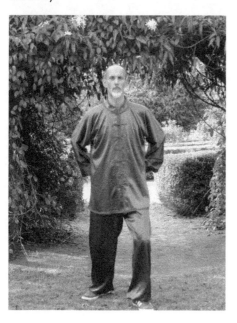

5 Shift the weight to the front leg, bend the right knee up, and get hold of the front of the knee with the right hand and the lateral side below the knee with the left hand (Stomach 37).

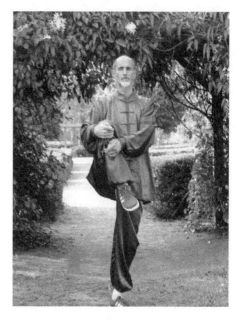

GOLDEN ROOSTER STANDS ON ONE LEG

6 Lower the right knee and step back with the right foot shifting the weight to the rear leg. At the same time, raise the hands up the sides of the body with the thumb and first finger held together and turn the head to the right side.

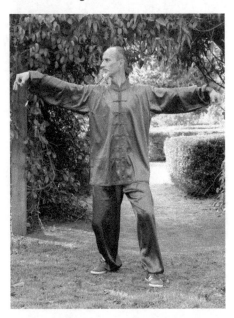

7 Bring the right foot forward parallel with the left foot. At the same time lower the hands down the sides to the *Dantian*.

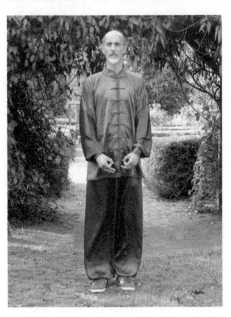

8 Repeat the exercise on the opposite side.

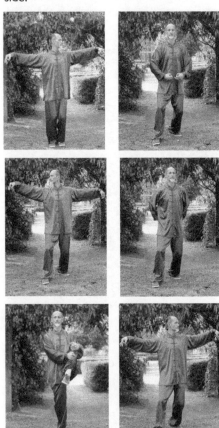

GOLDEN ROOSTER STANDS ON ONE LEG

Observations

‣ Maintain the shoulders lowered and relaxed.

‣ Hold the bending of the knee for about ten seconds.

Precautions and contraindications

This exercise may be contraindicated in cases of serious back conditions and severe dizziness.

Breathing method

Breathe in while raising the arms and when raising the knee. Breathe out while lowering the arms and when lowering the knee.

Flow of Qi

Lifting and bending up the knee stimulates the flow of Qi to the pelvic region and the large intestine. Standing on one leg activates the flow of Qi down the leg. Pressing on the leg below the knee stimulates Stomach 37, the lower uniting point of the large intestine Qi channel, thus promoting intestinal functions.

Mind focus

Focus on keeping the body upright, bending the knee up toward the chest, and coordinating the movement of the body with the breathing.

Main Qi channel

Large intestine.

Secondary Qi channels

Kidney, stomach.

Main benefits

‣ Compresses, stretches, and massages the abdomen, stimulating large intestine function.

‣ Tones up the intestines, improving bowel motility.

‣ Helps to balance the autonomic nervous system, thus regulating bowel function.

‣ Strengthens the leg and core muscles.

‣ Relieves abdominal pain, bloating, constipation, diarrhea, rumbling of the intestines, and difficult menses.

‣ Helps to ground the Qi, improving balance and mental focus.

Chapter 6

Daoist Yoga Exercises for the Stomach Energy Meridian

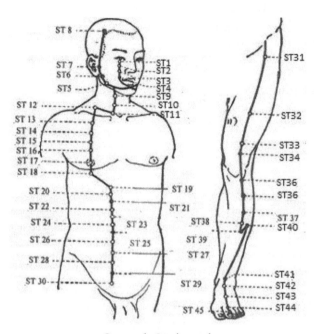

Stomach Qi channel

Pathway of the Qi channel

The stomach channel starts under the eye, moves down the face to the jaw area, and up in front of the ear to the corner of the forehead. From the jaw it runs down the throat and then moves out above the collar bone four inches from the midline of the body. The channel travels down the chest to below the breast area, then it moves in two inches from the anterior midline of the body and continues running down the upper and lower abdomen. From the pubic region it runs out over the lower abdomen and then moves down the leg following the anterior lateral aspect of the thigh, knee, and lower leg to the middle of the ankle joint. The channel continues down over the dorsum of the foot, ending at the lateral side of the second toe. The stomach channel has 45 vital points.

Internal branches

1. From under the eye a branch runs to the inner corner of the eye.

2. From the side of the nose a branch runs to the upper gums and around the lips.

3. From the corner of the forehead a branch runs to the midpoint of the forehead half an inch within the anterior hairline.

4. From the point above the collar bone a branch runs down the chest, crosses the diaphragm, enters into the stomach, and connects to the spleen. The internal path from the stomach travels down the lower abdomen and comes out at the point two inches lateral to the pubic bone.

5. From the lower leg (Stomach 40) a branch goes over the dorsum of the foot and then connects to the spleen channel at the big toe. Yet another branch departs three inches below the knee (Stomach 36) and runs parallel to the main channel to end at the lateral corner of the third toe.

Main signs of imbalance

Signs of excess (Fullness of Qi)

Stomach pain made worse by eating and pressure, fullness and discomfort of the upper abdomen, burning sensation in the upper abdomen, heartburn, acid reflux, sour or acid taste in the mouth, ulcers or blisters in the mouth, bad breath (halitosis), vomiting, burping or belching, hiccups, frontal headaches, pain and redness of the eyes, nosebleed, bleeding gums, excessive appetite, swelling and pain in the breast (mastitis), heat sensation on the anterior aspect of the body, manic depressive states, dark yellow urine, and pain in the lateral aspect of the lower limbs.

Signs of weakness (Emptiness of Qi)

Dull pain in the abdomen made worse on an empty stomach and improved by eating, sensation of coldness in the stomach region, difficulty ingesting foods, excess appetite without desire for eating, belching and burping, abdominal bloating, sensation of fullness during and after meals, lack of tone and mobility of the lower limbs, dry mouth, cold sensation on the anterior aspect of the body, difficulty digesting raw foods, and vomiting of clear fluid.

Main areas covered

Eyes, face, nose, upper gums, mouth, jaw, forehead, head, throat, chest, breasts, upper abdomen, stomach, spleen, pancreas, lower abdomen, anterior lateral aspect of thigh, lateral knee, anterior lateral aspect of lower leg, ankle joint, dorsum of foot, and second and third toes.

SEPARATING HEAVEN AND EARTH

Main vital points

Conception Vessel 12 (middle stomach) four inches above the navel, Urinary Bladder 21 (stomach transport) on the back, two fingers lateral from the 12th thoracic vertebra, Pericardium 8 (labored palace) on the center of the palm between the second and third metacarpal bones, Stomach 25 (celestial pivot) two inches lateral to the navel, Stomach 36 (leg three miles) four fingers below the inferior lateral border of the kneecap, Stomach 45 (severe mouth) at the lateral side of the second toe.

Main muscle groups

Anterior deltoid (anterior aspect of shoulder between lateral collar bone and upper arm), **coracobrachialis** (anterior medial aspect of upper arm), supinator (lateral superior aspect of forearm), pronator teres (anterior aspect of forearm across from medial elbow to middle of lateral radius bone), pronator quadratus (anterior aspect of forearm horizontally across proximal wrist), **pectoralis major** (chest region from chest bone and medial collar bone to upper arm), **biceps brachii** (anterior aspect of upper arm), **extensor carpi radialis brevis** (posterior aspect of forearm between lateral aspect of elbow and base of third finger), **external oblique** (lateral aspect of abdomen from lower 8 ribs to abdomen and crest of hip bone), **internal oblique** (lateral aspect of abdomen from anterior hip bone to lower 4 ribs and abdomen), **tensor fascia latae** (lateral aspect of thigh between crest of hip bone and lateral aspect of knee), **hamstrings** (posterior aspect of thigh between sitting bone and posterior knee), rectus abdominis (anterior aspect of abdomen between pubic bone and lower end of chest bone), transverse abdominis (horizontally across abdomen from lateral to medial), **extensor carpi radialis longus** (posterior aspect of forearm between lateral aspect of elbow and base of second finger).

Secondary muscle groups

Brachialis (anterior inferior aspect of upper arm between upper arm bone and ulna bone), **middle trapezius** (upper back area from thoracic vertebrae to spine of shoulder blade), pectoralis minor (chest region between anterior 3, 4, and 5 ribs and anterior shoulder blade), infraspinatus (shoulder blade region), teres minor (lateral inferior aspect of shoulder blade), abductor pollicis longus (posterior aspect of forearm from lower 2/3 to base of thumb).

Starting position

Stand with the feet shoulder-width apart and hands by the sides.

Description of the exercise

1 From the standing position bring both hands to the waist with the palms up.

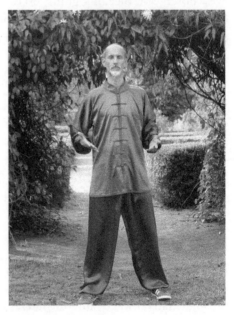

SEPARATING HEAVEN AND EARTH

2 Turn the body left, extending the right arm to the left side.

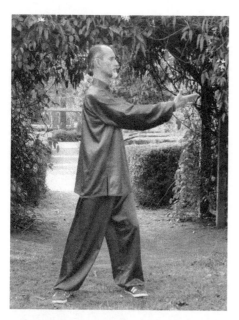

3 Turn right, extending the right arm to the right side with palm up.

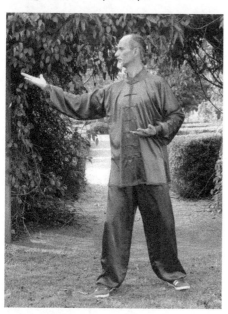

4 Continue turning to the right and back, bending the elbow, and rotating the wrist out with fingers pointing back and palm up.

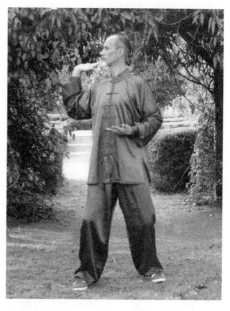

5 Stretch the right hand straight up above the head with fingers pointing to the left, and the left hand down the left side with fingers to front while breathing out. At the same time look at the lower hand.

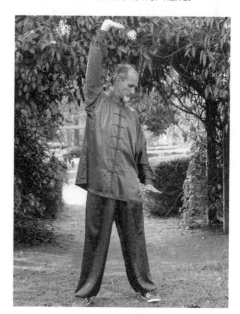

SEPARATING HEAVEN AND EARTH

6 Bend the right arm down behind the neck with palm facing down, and the left arm up to the mid-abdomen with palm facing up while breathing in.

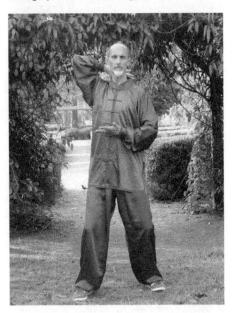

7 Extend the right arm up above the head with fingers pointing to left, and the left arm down with fingers pointing front while breathing out.

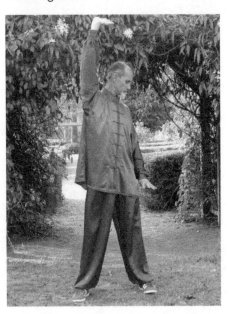

8 Bend and extend the arms one more time.

9 Turn right and bring the back of the left hand to the lower thoracic area (Urinary Bladder 21).

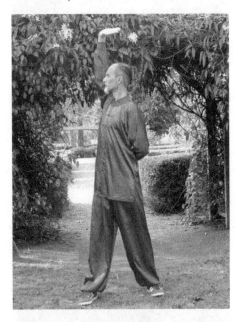

10 Turn left while breathing in.

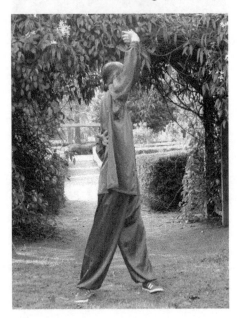

SEPARATING HEAVEN AND EARTH

11 Bend the body down the left side, moving the right palm down the face, throat, chest, abdomen, thigh, lower leg, and foot tracing the pathway of the stomach Qi channel while breathing out.

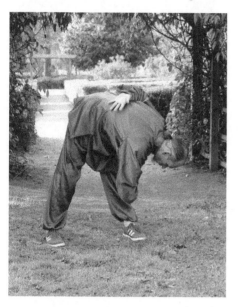

12 From the left foot move the right hand to the lateral side of the right foot, then bring the hand in between the two feet turning the palm up.

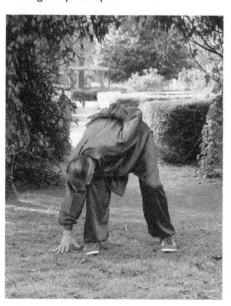

13 Slowly straighten up the body, bringing both hands back to the sides of the waist with palms up.

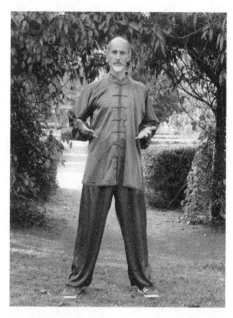

14 Repeat the same movement on the opposite side.

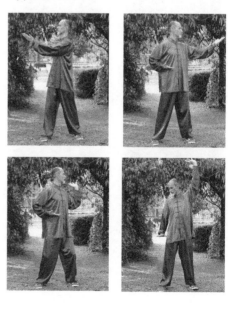

SEPARATING HEAVEN AND EARTH

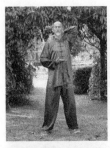
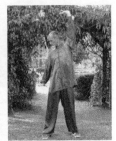
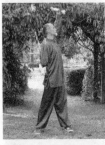
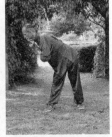
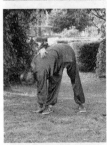
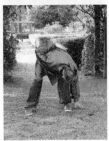
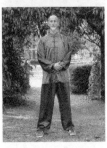

Observations

‣ When extending the hands up, turn the body slightly in the direction of the lower hand; and when flexing the hands, turn the body in the direction of the upper hand.

‣ When extending the hands, gaze at the lower hand, but maintain the head upright.

Precautions and contraindications

This exercise can be contraindicated in cases of slipped disc, serious back conditions, sciatica, high blood pressure, and vertigo.

Breathing method

Breathe in when flexing the arms, when turning the body before bending down the sides, and when straightening up the body. Breathe out when extending the hands and when bending the body down the sides.

Flow of Qi

When extending the hands to the head, Qi flows up and down the stomach meridian; when bending the body down, Qi flows down the face, chest, abdomen, thigh, leg, and foot along the stomach Qi channel.

Mind focus

When extending the hands, focus on stretching the chest and abdomen. When bending the body, focus on guiding the flow of Qi down along the stomach Qi channel.

Main Qi channel

Stomach.

SEPARATING HEAVEN AND EARTH

Secondary Qi channels

Large intestine, spleen, urinary bladder.

Main benefits

‣ Stretches the chest and abdominal muscle groups along the stomach Qi channel.

‣ Helps the ascending of the spleen Qi and descending of the stomach Qi, thus improving digestion.

‣ Stimulates the descending movement of Qi along the stomach channel, relieving nausea, vomiting, constipation, burping, and hiccups.

‣ Relaxes tightness of the diaphragm, soothing digestion.

‣ Provides a lateral stretch to the spine and the legs.

BRUSHING THE SHOELACES WITH THE HAND

Main vital points
Conception Vessel 12 (middle stomach), four inches above the navel, Pericardium 8 (labored palace) on the center of the palm between the second and third metacarpal bones, Stomach 25 (celestial pivot) two inches lateral to the navel, Stomach 36 (leg three miles) four fingers down from the inferior lateral aspect of the kneecap, Stomach 45 (severe mouth) on the lateral side of the second toe.

Main muscle groups
Biceps brachii (anterior aspect of upper arm), **coracobrachialis** (anterior medial aspect of upper arm), supinator (lateral superior aspect of forearm), anconeus (lateral aspect of shoulder), **extensor carpi radialis brevis** (posterior aspect of forearm between lateral aspect of elbow and base of third finger), **anterior deltoid** (anterior aspect of shoulder between lateral collar bone and upper arm), supraspinatus (superior aspect of shoulder blade), **external oblique** (lateral aspect of abdomen from lower 8 ribs to abdomen and crest of hip bone), **internal oblique** (lateral aspect of abdomen from anterior hip bone to lower 4 ribs and abdomen), **tensor fascia latae** (lateral aspect of thigh between crest of hip bone and lateral aspect of knee), **rectus abdominis** (anterior aspect of abdomen between pubic bone and lower end of chest bone), **transversospinalis multifidus** (along spine from transverse processes of vertebrae to spinous processes of vertebrae spanning 2 to 4 vertebrae segments), **transversospinalis rotators** (spine between transverse processes of vertebrae and spinous processes of vertebra directly above), **pectoralis major** (chest region from chest bone and medial collar bone to upper arm).

Secondary muscle groups
Brachialis (anterior inferior aspect of upper arm between upper arm bone and ulna bone), triceps (posterior aspect of upper arm between upper arm and elbow), pronator quadratus (anterior aspect of forearm horizontally across proximal wrist), pronator teres (anterior aspect of forearm across from medial elbow to middle of lateral radius bone), quadratum lumborum (lower back area from posterior hip bone to lumbar vertebrae and 12th rib).

Starting position
Stand with the feet together and hands by the sides.

Description of the exercise

1 Bring the right hand level with the navel with the palm facing up and the left hand level with the chest with the palm down as if holding a ball. Focus on the sensation of Qi between the hands.

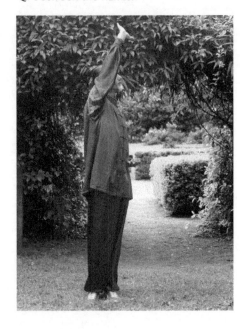

BRUSHING THE SHOELACES WITH THE HAND

2 Move the right hand out and straight up above the head with the palm facing up and fingers pointing to left, and the left hand down to the left side of the waist with palm up. At the same time turn the body to the left.

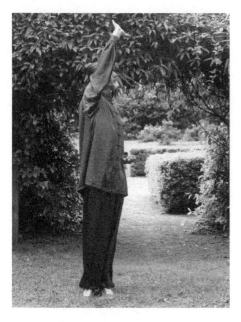

3 First turn the body right and then turn it left as you breathe in.

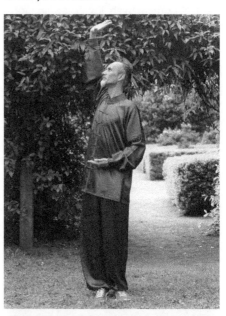

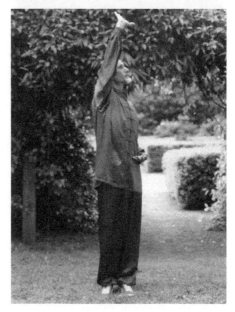

BRUSHING THE SHOELACES WITH THE HAND

4 Bend the body down the left side, moving the right palm down the face, chest, abdomen, thigh, lower leg, and foot tracing the pathway of the stomach Qi channel. At the same time breathe out.

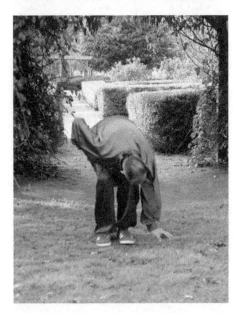

5 Turn the right hand around to the right side and making a loose fist grab Qi from earth.

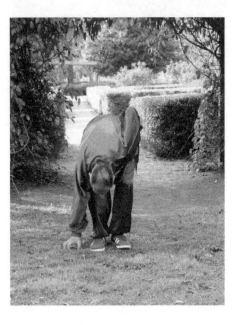

6 Straightening the body bring the right hand up to the right side of the waist as you breathe in. The right hand ends resting on the waist in a loose fist. In a continuous movement bring the left hand straight up the centerline of the body, all the way above the head with the palm facing up and fingers pointing right. At the same time turn the body to the right.

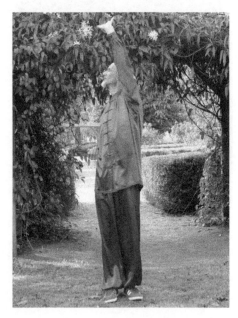

BRUSHING THE SHOELACES WITH THE HAND

7 First turn the body left and then turn it right as you breathe in.

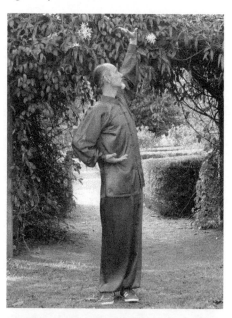

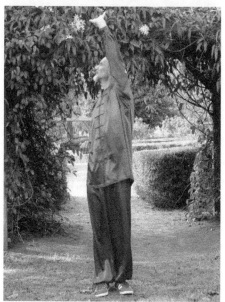

8 Bend the body down the right side moving the left palm along the face, chest, abdomen, thigh, lower leg, and foot tracing the path of the stomach Qi channel. At the same time breathe out.

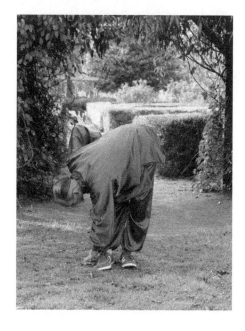

BRUSHING THE SHOELACES WITH THE HAND

9 Turn the left hand around to the left side and making a loose fist grab Qi from the earth, then straightening up the body bring the hand up to the left side of the waist as you breathe in. The left hand ends resting on the waist in a loose fist.

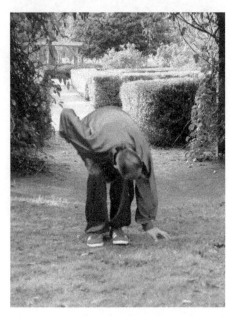

10 Continue the exercise down the left and right sides of the body for several times.

11 End the exercise by bringing the hands to the lower *Dantian*.

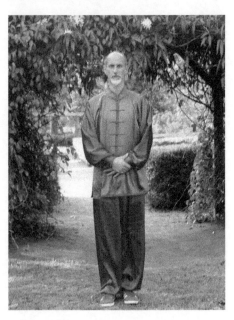

Observations

▸ Initially bend the body down the sides slowly and then bend the body more quickly.

▸ Coordinate the movements of the body with the breathing.

▸ When bending down the body keep the hips stable.

Precautions and contraindications

This exercise is contraindicated for people suffering from heart disease, high blood pressure, slipped disc, serious back conditions, sciatica, hernia, and vertigo.

BRUSHING THE SHOELACES WITH THE HAND

Breathing method

Breathe in when straightening up the body and lifting up the hand. Breathe out when bending the body down and lowering the hand.

Flow of Qi

When extending the hand above the head, Qi flows up the abdomen, chest, and face. When bending the body, Qi flows down the face, trunk, and leg along the stomach Qi channel.

Mind focus

Focus on turning the body from the waist, bending down from the hips, keeping the hips and pelvis stable when bending the body down and coordinating the movements with the breathing.

Main Qi channel

Stomach.

Secondary Qi channels

Spleen, kidney, urinary bladder, conception vessel (*Ren Mai*).

Main benefits

‣ Same as the exercise above.

‣ Increases flexibility of the back and legs.

‣ Helps to reduce excess weight around the waist.

Chapter 7

Daoist Yoga Exercises for the Spleen Energy Meridian

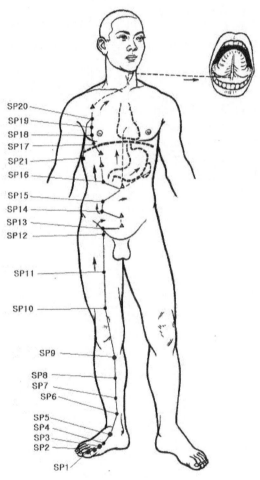

SP20
SP19
SP18
SP17
SP21
SP16

SP15
SP14
SP13
SP12

SP11

SP10

SP9

SP8
SP7
SP6

SP5
SP4
SP3
SP2

SP1

Spleen Qi channel

Pathway of the Qi channel

The spleen channel starts from the medial side of the big toe, moves over the arch of the foot, and up in front of the inner ankle bone. The channel continues up the anterior medial aspect of the lower leg just posterior to the tibia (shin bone), travels through the medial side of the knee, and up the anterior medial aspect of the thigh to the lower abdomen. It then runs up the lower and upper abdomen four inches lateral from the anterior midline of the body, and continues further up the ribs and out the second intercostal space six inches from the midline of the body. The channel then moves down the side of the trunk, ending at the side of the ribs. This channel has 21 vital points along its course.

Internal branches

1. From the upper thigh the channel moves into the lower abdomen and the reproductive organs.

2. From the point four inches lateral to the navel (Spleen 15) an internal branch travels to the spleen and connects to the stomach.

3. From the stomach a branch flows up into the heart.

4. From the uppermost point on the chest (Spleen 20) a branch runs up passing alongside the esophagus, connects to the root of the tongue, and spreads over its lower surface.

5. From the last point on the chest the foot spleen greater Yin channel connects to the hand lung greater Yin channel.

Main signs of imbalance

Signs of excess (Fullness of Qi)

Abdominal bloating or distension, sensation of heaviness in the abdomen, nausea, vomiting, abdominal pain, mucus congestion and excessive mucus discharge, mucus in the stool, excess weight especially on the mid-abdomen, waist, hips and thighs, pain, tenderness, or soreness under the rib cage on the left side of the abdomen, sluggishness and heaviness of the body, damp and clammy skin, symptoms made worse by humid weather, sensation of a lump in the abdomen, excessive gas, jaundice (yellow discoloration of the skin, eyes, palms and feet), rigidity of the tongue, over-concerned and obsessive behavior, and pain and spasm of the feet.

Signs of weakness (Emptiness of Qi)

Sallow facial complexion (pale-yellow face), weak digestion, poor appetite, anorexia, poor assimilation and absorption of nutrients, low energy and fatigue, abdominal bloating and indigestion long after eating, loose stools or diarrhea, craving for sweets, dull pain in the abdomen alleviated by heat, low body weight, rumbling of the intestines (borborygmus), nausea, cold limbs, bruising easily (capillary fragility), poor muscle tone, flaccid flesh, weakness and lack of tone of the extremities, sensation of cold along the inner aspect of the legs, edema of the legs, sagging (prolapse) of internal organs and tissues, prolapsed rectum or uterus, excessive uterine bleeding with light red blood profuse in amount (functional uterine bleeding), and excessive worry and anxiety.

Main areas covered

Big toe, medial border of foot, anterior aspect of ankle, anterior medial aspect of lower leg, medial aspect of knee, anterior medial aspect of thigh, groin, lower abdomen, reproductive organs, middle abdomen, spleen, pancreas, stomach, upper abdomen, heart, lungs, lateral aspect of chest, rib side, armpit, esophagus, root of tongue, and lower surface of tongue.

EARTH CLOUDS

Main vital points

Pericardium 8 (labored palace) on the center of the palm between the second and third metacarpal bones, *Dantian* (elixir field) 3 inches below the navel, Conception Vessel 17 (middle of the breasts) on the center of the chest between the breasts, Spleen 21 (great connecting) at the side of the ribs halfway between the middle of the armpit and the eleventh free rib, Liver 13 (bright door) below the eleventh rib, Gall Bladder 26 on the side of the waist level with the navel and on line with the eleventh rib, Stomach 25 (celestial pivot) 2 inches lateral to the navel.

Main muscle groups

Biceps brachii (anterior aspect of upper arm), **latissimus dorsi** (from crest of hip bone, sacrum, and lower thoracic vertebrae across lower and middle back to posterior aspect of upper arm), anterior deltoid (anterior superior aspect of the shoulder), **middle deltoid** (superior lateral aspect of shoulder), supraspinatus (superior aspect of shoulder blade), infraspinatus (on shoulder blade region), coracobrachialis (medial aspect of upper arm), **external oblique** (lateral abdomen from lower eight ribs to abdomen and crest of hip), **intercostals** (between adjacent ribs), iliopsoas (deep abdominal region from lumbar vertebrae to inner superior aspect of femur), **rectus femoris** (on the anterior aspect of the thigh).

Secondary muscle groups

Posterior deltoid (posterior aspect of the shoulder from inferior spine of shoulder blade to upper arm bone), **pectoralis major** (chest region), rectus abdominis (on abdomen from pubic bone to lower end of chest bone), internal oblique (lateral inferior abdomen from groin area and crest of hip to lower fourth rib and abdomen), quadratus lumborum (lower back area from posterior hip to lower fourth vertebrae and twelfth rib).

Starting position

Stand with the feet slightly wider than the shoulders with hands by the sides.

Description of the exercise

1 Step in with the right foot, turn the waist to the left and transfer the weight onto the left leg. At the same time, bring the right hand up level with the chest, palm facing down and the left hand down level with the lower abdomen palm facing up, like holding a ball.

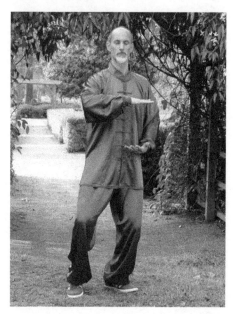

EARTH CLOUDS

2 Stepping out with the right foot, turn the waist to the right and transfer the weight onto the right leg with the hands holding a ball.

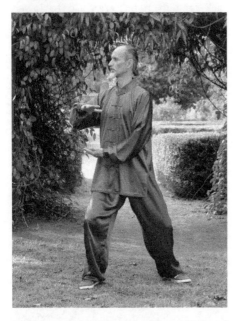

3 Rotate the ball bringing the right hand down level with the lower abdomen with palm facing up and the left hand up level with the chest with palm facing down.

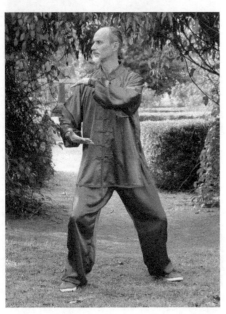

4 Turn the waist to the left shifting the weight onto the left leg with the hands holding a ball.

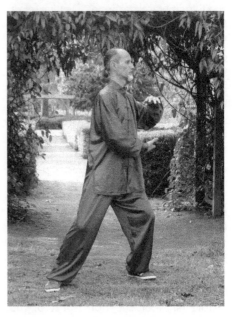

5 Rotate the ball bringing the right hand up level with the chest with palm facing down and the left hand down level with the lower abdomen with palm facing up.

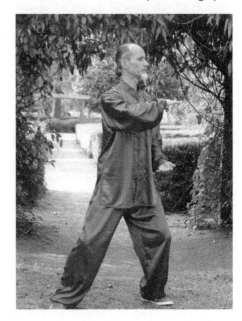

EARTH CLOUDS

6 Shift weight onto the right leg stepping in with the left foot. At the same time bring the right hand down inferior to the eleventh rib and the left hand up level with the face.

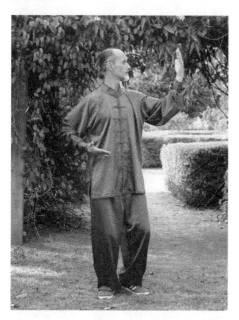

7 Extend the left hand out to the left side with fingers facing to the front and palm facing out. At the same time lift the right knee and look at the left palm.

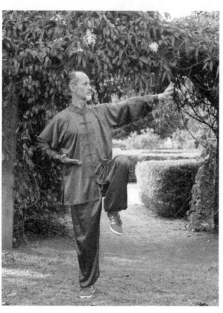

8 Lower the left hand to above the left shoulder at the same time lowering the right leg and slightly bending both knees.

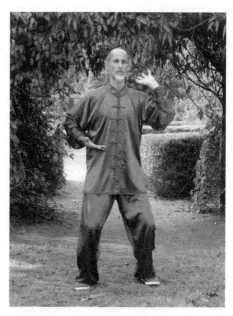

9 Extend the left hand all the way up rotating the palm in to face back.

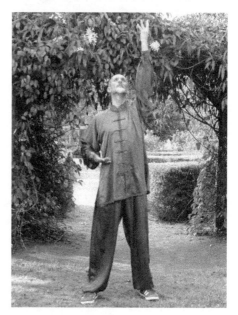

EARTH CLOUDS

10 Rotate the left hand out to face the front and lower the hand to the lower abdomen joining with the right hand at the lower *Dantian*.

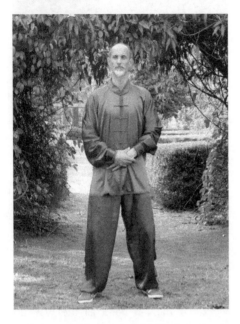

11 Repeat the exercise on the opposite side.

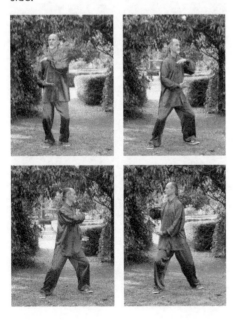

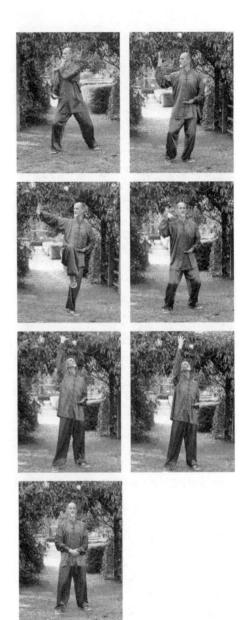

EARTH CLOUDS

Observations

‣ Focus on turning the body from the waist and abdomen and not just the shoulders or hips.

‣ When rotating the ball in the hands follow the flow of Qi around the abdomen.

Precautions and contraindications

When bending the knee, lift the knee only as far as it is comfortable and safe.

Breathing technique

Breathe in when rotating the ball, when moving the hand up in front of the face, and when bringing the hand above the shoulder. Breathe out when turning the body to the sides, when extending the hand out to the side, and when stretching the hand up above the head.

Flow of Qi

Qi flows left and right around the abdomen, out to the side of the body from the ribs, and up and down the front of the body.

Mind focus

Focus the mind on turning from the waist, rotating the abdomen, and the flow of Qi around the abdomen and up and down the body.

Main Qi channels

Spleen-pancreas, stomach.

Secondary Qi channels

Liver, gall bladder, kidney.

Main benefits

‣ Stimulates digestion and assimilation of food.

‣ Improves appetite.

‣ Helps to relieve indigestion, poor appetite, abdominal distention, nausea, chest congestion, acid reflux, diarrhea, low energy, and edema.

‣ Activates the flow of vital energy or Qi in the abdomen and the waist supporting spleen, liver, gall bladder, stomach, and pancreatic functions.

‣ Promotes intestinal mobility and regularity.

THE GREAT SWALLOW FLYING
OVER THE NEST

Main vital points

Pericardium 8 (labored palace) on the center of the palm between the second and third metacarpal bones, Liver 13 (bright door) below the eleventh rib, Urinary Bladder 20 (spleen transport) on the back, two fingers lateral to the eleventh thoracic vertebra, Spleen 21 (great connecting) on the side of the ribs, Large Intestine 15 (shoulder bone) lateral anterior to the shoulder joint.

Main muscle groups

Biceps brachii (anterior aspect of upper arm), **pectoralis major** (chest region from chest bone and medial collar bone to upper arm), anterior deltoid (anterior aspect of shoulder between lateral collar bone and upper arm), **posterior deltoid** (posterior aspect of shoulder between shoulder blade and upper arm), **latissimus dorsi** (from crest of hip bone, sacrum, and lower thoracic vertebrae across middle and lower back to posterior aspect of upper arm), supraspinatus (superior aspect of shoulder blade), quadratum lumborum (lower back area from posterior hip bone to lumbar vertebrae and 12th rib), **external oblique** (lateral aspect of abdomen from lower 8 ribs to abdomen and hip bone), **internal oblique** (lateral aspect of abdomen from anterior hip bone to lower 4 ribs and abdomen), teres major (from inferior angle of shoulder blade to medial aspect of upper arm), triceps (posterior aspect of upper arm between upper arm and elbow), **intercostals** (between ribs).

Secondary muscle groups

Upper trapezius (neck and shoulder region between neck vertebrae and lateral aspect of collar bone), lower trapezius (middle back between thoracic vertebrae and root of spine of shoulder blade), erector spinae (along back between vertebrae, posterior ribs, and occipital bone), intertransversarii (between transverse processes of vertebrae), **flexor carpi ulnaris** (posterior medial aspect of forearm, between lateral elbow and base of fifth finger), flexor carpi radialis (anterior aspect of forearm, between lateral elbow and bases of second and third fingers), pectoralis minor (chest region between anterior 3, 4, and 5 ribs and anterior shoulder blade).

Starting position

Step out into a middle-height horse-riding stance with the feet apart about twice the width of the shoulders.

Description of the exercise

1 Place the hands at the waist with palms up.

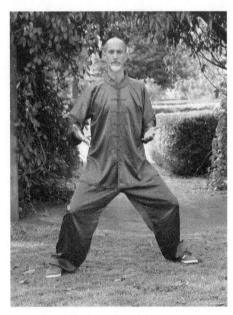

THE GREAT SWALLOW FLYING
OVER THE NEST

2 Turn the body to the left side extending the right hand horizontally to the left side as you shift the weight to the left leg and breathe out.

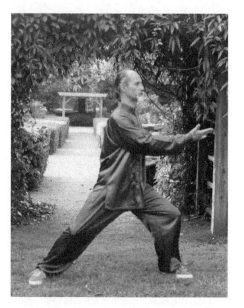

3 Turn the body to the right side extending the right hand horizontally to the right side as you shift the weight to the right leg and breathe in.

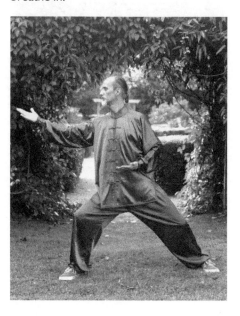

4 Bend the body sideways to the left side shifting the weight to the left leg and stretching the right arm up and over to the left side. At the same time, move the left hand across to the right side under the eleventh rib while breathing out.

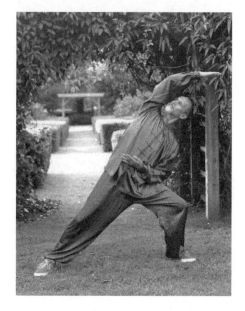

THE GREAT SWALLOW FLYING
OVER THE NEST

5 Rotate the right hand in under the right armpit and down the trunk, extending the hand out to the right side turning the palm up. At the same time shift the weight to the right leg.

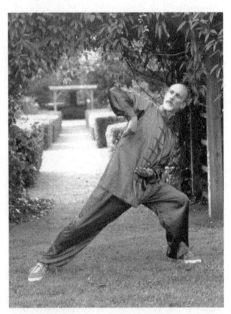

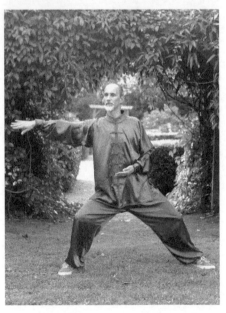

6 Rotate the right hand medially toward the front of the abdomen, shifting the weight to the left leg and breathing in.

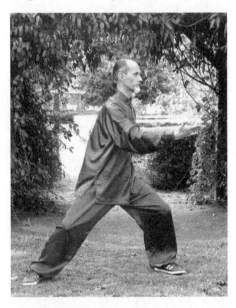

7 Turn the body to the right side extending the left hand horizontally to the right side as you shift the weight to the right leg and breathe out.

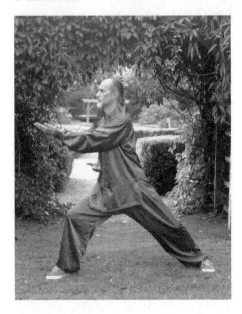

THE GREAT SWALLOW FLYING
OVER THE NEST

8 Turn the body to the left side extending the left hand horizontally to the left side as you shift the weight to the left leg and breathe in.

9 Bend the body to the right side shifting the weight to the right leg and stretching the left arm up and over to the right side. At the same time, move the right hand across to the left side under the eleventh rib while breathing out.

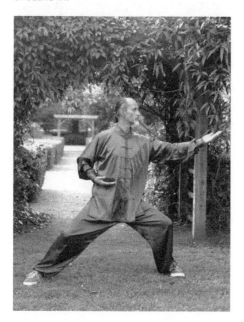

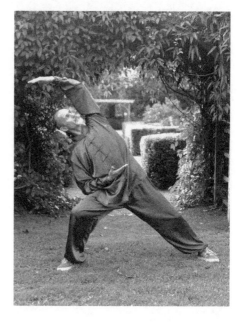

THE GREAT SWALLOW FLYING OVER THE NEST

10 Rotate the left hand in under the left armpit and down the trunk, extending the hand out to the left side. At the same time shift the weight to the left leg.

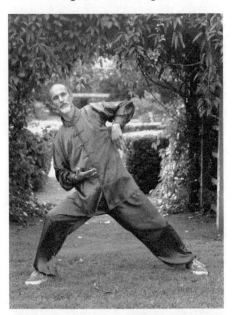

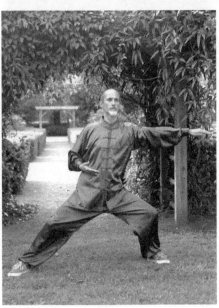

11 Rotate the left hand medially toward the front of the abdomen, shifting the weight to the right leg and breathing in.

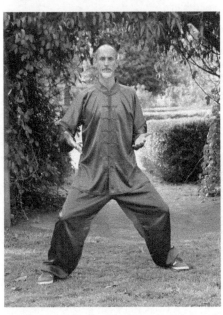

12 Alternate the movement turning to the left and right sides several times.

13 Finish the exercise by bringing both hands to the lower abdomen.

Observations

- When shifting weight, pay attention to bending the knee in the direction of the toes and keeping the hips facing square to the front.

- Avoid bending the knee past beyond the toes.

- Alternate turning to the left and right sides several times.

THE GREAT SWALLOW FLYING
OVER THE NEST

Breathing method

Breathe out when first turning the body to the side and breathe in when turning to the opposite side. Breathe out again when bending the body sideways and extending the hand over the head, and breathe in when bringing the hands to the lower abdomen.

Flow of Qi

Qi flows side to side horizontally in the abdomen and along the spleen Qi channel.

Mind focus

Focus on the movement of Qi along the abdomen and ribs side, and coordinating the movements with the breathing.

Main Qi channel

Spleen.

Secondary Qi channels

Liver, gall bladder, small intestine.

Main benefits

‣ Turning and bending the trunk stimulates the flow of Qi in the abdomen.

‣ Works out the mid-back, lower back, shoulder, ribs, and abdominal muscle groups associated with the spleen Qi channel.

‣ Relieves indigestion, fullness of the abdomen, pain in the ribs, chest congestion, and fluid retention in the abdomen.

‣ Helps condition the abdomen, waist, ribs, shoulder, back, and leg muscles.

Chapter 8

Daoist Yoga Exercises for the Heart Energy Meridian

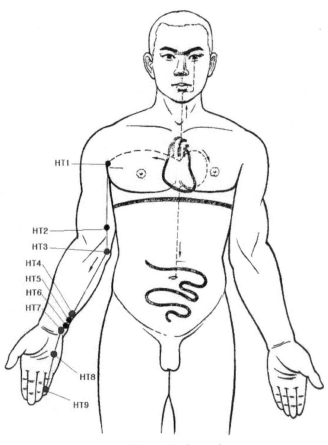

Heart Qi channel

Pathway of the Qi channel

The heart channel starts from the heart, travels across the chest and comes out to the surface of the body at the center of the armpit. It then moves down the anterior medial aspect of the upper arm, the elbow, and the lower arm to reach the inner side of the wrist. It continues over the palm between the fourth and fifth fingers ending at the lateral or thumb side of the little finger. The heart channel has nine vital points.

Internal branches

1. One branch travels from the heart downward through the diaphragm and connects to the small intestine.

2. A second branch comes out of the heart, moves up along the esophagus, rises up to the eyes, and continues upward to connect to the brain.

3. A further branch moves up across the chest region connecting with the lungs and coming out at the armpit.

Main signs of imbalance

Signs of excess (Fullness of Qi)

Cardiac pain which may radiate to the shoulder, neck, and arm, sensation of fullness and pain in the chest, chest discomfort when lying down, pain in the ribs and hypochondriac region, palpitations, insomnia, mental restlessness, dream-disturbed sleep, nightmares, flushed face, thirst, ulcers or sores and pain in the mouth and tongue, hot or painful palms, pain in the shoulder blade region, pain along the course of the Qi channel, incoherent speech, excessive talking, mental disorders, aggressive and violent behavior, and red tongue especially at the tip.

Signs of weakness (Emptiness of Qi)

Palpitations, shortness of breath that is made worse by exertion, weakness and fatigue, spontaneous sweating, weak pulse or missed beat pulse, poor circulation, cold extremities in particular the hands, pale facial complexion, poor memory, insomnia with difficulty falling asleep or waking up at night, dizziness with fainting spells, dryness of the mouth, inability to speak, pale tongue, night sweating and mental restlessness.

Main areas covered

Heart, chest, lungs, armpit, anterior medial aspect of upper arm, elbow and forearm, little finger side of palm, little finger, small intestine, esophagus, eyes, and brain.

INVIGORATING THE HEART AND GUIDING QI

Main vital points

Conception Vessel 17 (middle of the breasts) on the center of the chest, Urinary Bladder 23 (kidney transport) on the lower back level with the second lumbar vertebra, Pericardium 8 (labored palace) on the center of the palm between the second and third metacarpal bones, Pericardium 9 (central hub) in the center of the tip of the middle finger, Heart 9 (lesser surge) on the inner side of the small finger.

Main muscle groups

Anterior deltoid (anterior aspect of shoulder between lateral collar bone and upper arm), pectoralis major (chest region from chest bone and medial collar bone to upper arm), triceps (posterior aspect of upper arm between upper arm and elbow), **biceps brachii** (anterior aspect of upper arm), coracobrachialis (anterior medial aspect of upper arm), infraspinatus (shoulder blade region), **supinator** (lateral superior aspect of forearm), teres major (from inferior angle of shoulder blade to medial aspect of upper arm), **pronator teres** (anterior aspect of forearm across from medial elbow to middle of lateral radius bone), extensor carpi radialis longus (posterior aspect of forearm between lateral aspect of elbow and base of second finger), extensor carpi radialis brevis (posterior aspect of forearm between lateral aspect of elbow and base of third finger), extensor carpi ulnaris (posterior aspect of forearm between lateral aspect of elbow and base of fifth finger), opponens digiti minimi (on palmar surface of fifth metacarpal finger), opponens pollicis (on palmar surface of thumb).

Secondary muscle groups

Middle deltoid (lateral superior aspect of upper arm), subscapularis (anterior aspect of shoulder blade), **posterior deltoid** (posterior aspect of shoulder between shoulder blade and upper arm), flexors of fingers (palm and dorsum of hand and palmar aspect of fingers), **serratus anterior** (chest wall between upper 8 ribs and anterior surface of shoulder blade), pectoralis minor (chest region between anterior 3, 4, and 5 ribs and anterior shoulder blade).

Starting position

Stand with the feet shoulder-width apart and knees slightly bent.

Description of the exercise

1 Bring the palms together in front of the chest in the Buddha or prayer palms position.

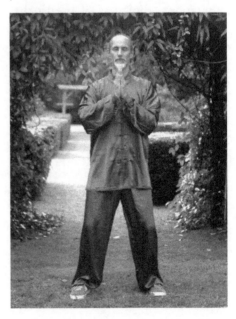

INVIGORATING THE HEART AND GUIDING QI

2 Hold this position for a few moments centering the Qi in the heart region.

3 Slowly rotate the hands out and down the sides toward the back of the body as you breathe out. End with palms down and fingers pointing to the front. Focus the mind on the kidney area.

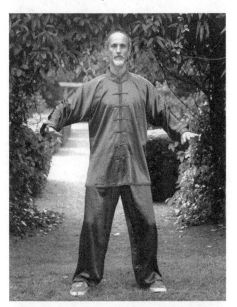

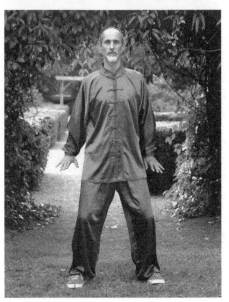

4 Turn the palms up, lifting the hands up and out in front of the body to chest level, focusing the intention on the tip of the middle fingers. At the same time breathe in.

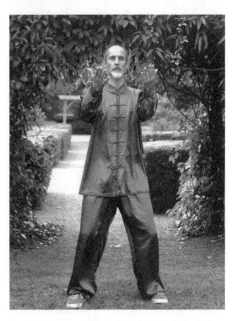

5 Rotate the hands in turning the palms down, focusing on the midpoint at the fleshy part of the thumb as you breathe out.

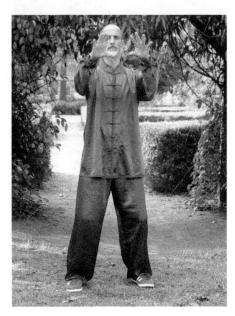

INVIGORATING THE HEART AND GUIDING QI

6 Make loose fists as if grabbing with the hands while breathing in.

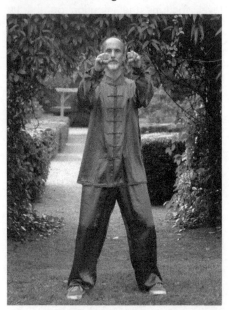

7 Bring the hands down the sides of the body as if pulling a heavy load while breathing out. End with the hands behind the body with loose fists.

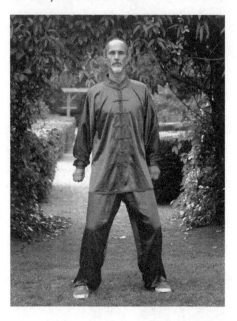

8 Focusing on the right hand turn the palm up, lifting the hand in front of the chest while breathing in.

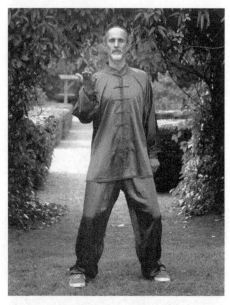

9 Turn the right palm out and push the hand to the front while breathing out. Focus on the center of the palm and the tips of the middle and little fingers.

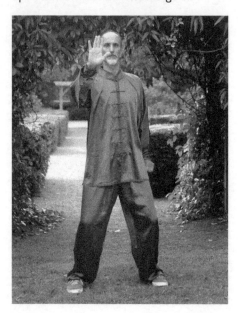

INVIGORATING THE HEART AND GUIDING QI

10 Bring the right hand back in front of the chest while breathing in.

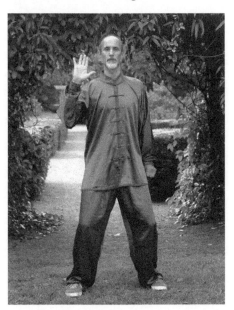

11 Turn the right palm down and move the hand down the side while breathing out.

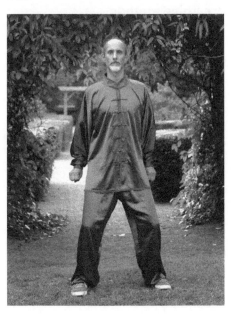

12 Focusing on the left hand, turn the palm up, lifting the hand in front of the chest while breathing in.

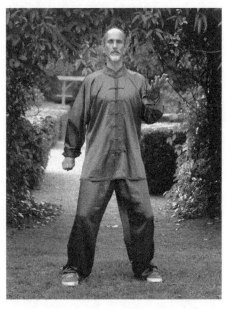

13 Turn the left palm out and push to the front while breathing out. Focus on the center of the palm and the tips of the middle and little fingers.

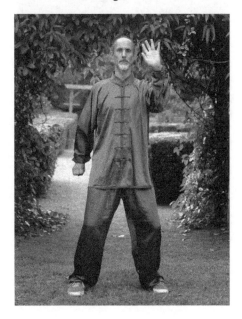

INVIGORATING THE HEART AND GUIDING QI

14 Bring the left hand back in front of the chest while breathing in.

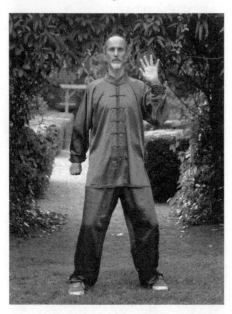

15 Turn the left palm down and lower the hand to the side of the body while breathing out.

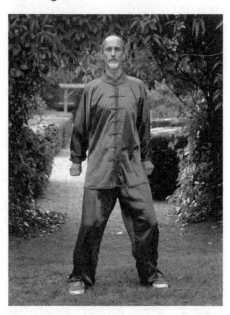

16 Bring both hands back to the chest in the Buddha or prayer palms position.

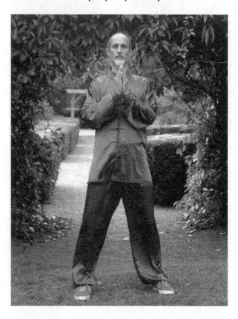

17 Repeat the exercise two or more times.

Breathing method
Breathe in when lifting and drawing back the hands. Breathe out when lowering and pushing out the hands.

Flow of Qi
Qi coordinates with the movement of the hands flowing from the heart down to the kidneys, up to the chest, out from the inner aspect of the arms to the center of the palms, and further to the tips of the middle and small fingers. It then flows back to the chest and down to the kidneys and lower *Dantian*.

Main Qi channel
Heart.

Secondary Qi channels
Pericardium, lung.

INVIGORATING THE HEART AND GUIDING QI

Main benefits

‣ Promotes the flow of Qi and blood through the heart channel.

‣ Helps to relieve palpitations, tightness in the chest, high blood pressure, irregular heartbeat, and nervous disorders.

‣ Calms the mind and relaxes the nerves in cases of insomnia, nervousness, stress, and sleep disorders.

‣ Helps to balance the energies of the kidneys (water) and the heart (fire), thus regulating the heart function.

NINE GHOSTS DRAWING A SABER

Main vital points

Urinary Bladder 15 (heart transport) on the upper back two fingers lateral to the fifth thoracic vertebra, Urinary Bladder 44 (spirit hall) three inches lateral to the fifth thoracic vertebra, Conception Vessel 17 (middle of the breasts) on the center of the chest, Heart 3 (lesser sea) on the medial aspect of the elbow at the end of the medial elbow crease, Heart 7 (spirit gate) on the little finger side of the wrist crease.

Main muscle groups

Anterior deltoid (anterior aspect of shoulder between lateral collar bone and upper arm), supraspinatus (superior aspect of shoulder blade), **upper trapezius** (neck and shoulder region between neck vertebrae and lateral aspect of collar bone), **posterior deltoid** (posterior aspect of shoulder between shoulder blade and upper arm), biceps brachii (anterior aspect of upper arm), **coracobrachialis** (anterior medial aspect of upper arm), **flexor digitorum profundus** (anterior aspect of forearm, hand, and fingers), flexor digitorum superficialis (anterior aspect of forearm and hand), **rhomboids** (shoulder blade area from thoracic vertebrae to medial border of shoulder blade), **serratus anterior** (chest wall between upper 8 ribs and anterior surface of shoulder blade), **pectoralis minor** (chest region between anterior 3, 4, and 5 ribs and anterior shoulder blade), **infraspinatus** (shoulder blade region), teres minor (lateral inferior aspect of shoulder blade), external oblique (lateral aspect of abdomen from lower 8 ribs to abdomen and crest of hip bone), internal oblique (lateral aspect of abdomen from anterior hip bone to lower 4 ribs and abdomen), rectus abdominis (anterior aspect of abdomen between pubic bone and lower end of chest bone), spinalis (cervical and thoracic vertebrae), transversospinalis multifidus (along spine from transverse processes of vertebrae to spinous processes of vertebrae spanning 2 to 4 vertebral segments).

Secondary muscle groups

Pectoralis major (chest region from chest bone and medial collar bone to upper arm), brachialis (anterior inferior aspect of upper arm between upper arm bone and ulna bone), middle deltoid (lateral superior aspect of upper arm), triceps (posterior aspect of upper arm between upper arm and elbow), teres major (from inferior angle of shoulder blade to medial aspect of upper arm).

Starting position

Stand with the feet slightly wider than the hips and hands by the sides.

Description of the exercise

1 Raise the arms up the sides to shoulder level.

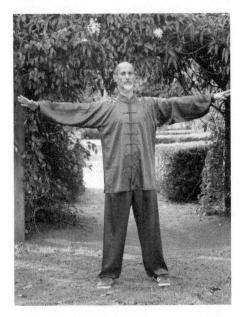

NINE GHOSTS DRAWING A SABER

2 Turn the body to the left, extending the right arm straight up above the head, and lowering the left arm down.

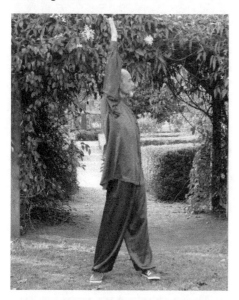

3 Turn the body to the right, bringing the dorsum of the left hand up behind the back and bending the right arm down with the palm facing the body. Interlock the hands behind the back, raising the right elbow and opening the right armpit, and closing in the left elbow and armpit. At the same time breathe in.

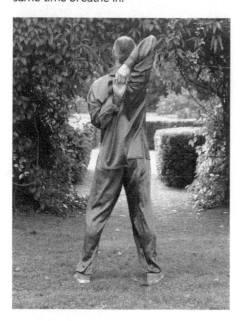

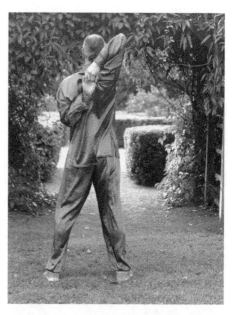

4 If unable to interlock the hands behind the back, bend the arms behind the back only as far as possible. One can also place the upper hand behind the head with the fingertips covering the top of the ear and the palm supporting the upper neck, or make use of a strap or a wooden *Taiji* stick to connect the hands behind the back.

NINE GHOSTS DRAWING A SABER

5 Bend the upper body down slightly toward the left side as drawing-in the right elbow, rounding the upper back area and bending the knees. At the same time breathe out.

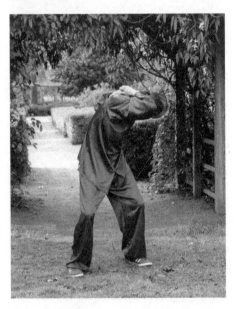

6 Straighten the back and turn the upper body slightly to the right, opening the right elbow and right armpit. At the same time look up breathing in.

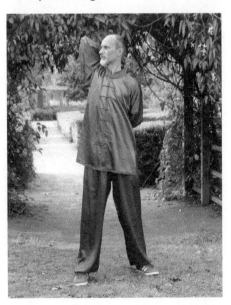

7 Bend and stretch the upper back two times more.

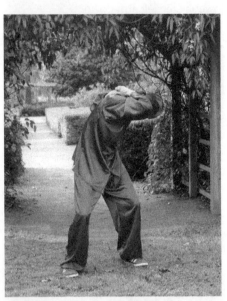

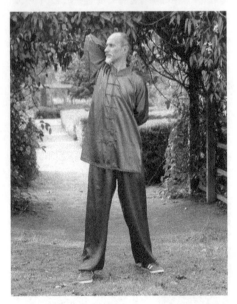

NINE GHOSTS DRAWING A SABER

8 Release the grab of the hands, extending the arms out at the sides. At the same time turn the body to the right extending the left arm straight up above the head and lowering the right arm down.

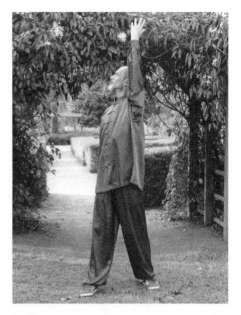

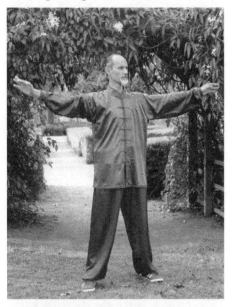

9 Turn left bringing the dorsum of the right hand up behind the back and the left hand down with the palm facing the body. Interlock the hands behind the back or the head.

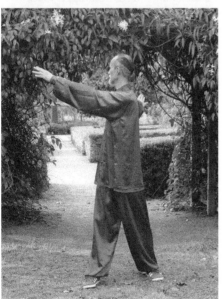

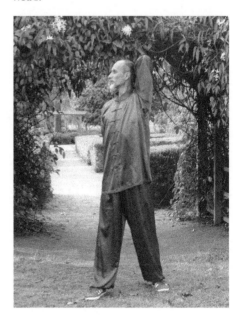

NINE GHOSTS DRAWING A SABER

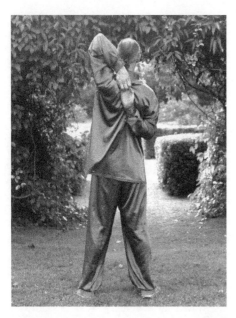

10 Bend the upper trunk down slightly toward the right as drawing-in the left elbow, rounding the upper back area and bending the knees. At the same time breathe out.

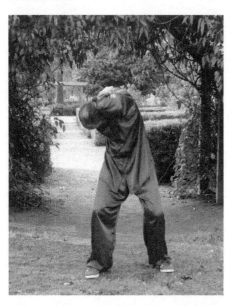

11 Straighten up the back and turn the upper body slightly to the left, opening the left elbow and left armpit. At the same time look up breathing in.

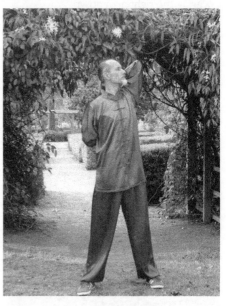

12 Bend and stretch the upper back two more times.

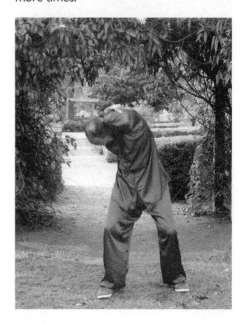

NINE GHOSTS DRAWING A SABER

13 Release the hands and lower the hands to the *Dantian*.

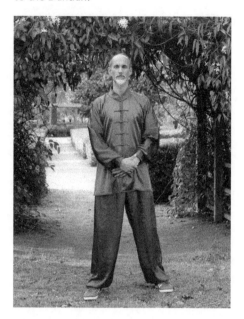

Observations

‣ When bending and straightening the back, focus the mind on extending out and opening the upper elbow and armpit while closing in the lower elbow and armpit.

‣ Throughout the exercise pay attention to maintaining the neck aligned with the spine.

‣ Keep the body weight even when bending and stretching the back.

Precautions and contraindications

This exercise may be contraindicated for people with severe neck conditions, painful conditions of the shoulders and arms, and high blood pressure.

Breathing method

Breathe in when straightening up the body. Breathe out when bending the body down.

Flow of Qi

Qi flows up and down the spine over the shoulder blade region and along the heart and small intestine Qi channels.

Mind focus

Focus on lengthening and bending the upper spine, opening and closing the chest, maintaining the spine and neck aligned, and coordinating the movements with the breathing.

Main Qi channel

Heart.

Secondary Qi channels

Small intestine, governing vessel (*Du Mai*).

Main benefits

‣ Releases tightness of the shoulder blades and upper back area.

‣ Calms the emotions and relieves nervous tension.

‣ Flexes and stretches the shoulder blades, chest, and shoulders, stimulating the main reflex areas associated with the heart.

‣ Stimulates the lung and heart functions, alleviating chest pain, cough, and asthma.

‣ Stimulates important vital points on the arms and hands, promoting the flow of Qi along the heart energy channel.

‣ Activates Qi and blood circulation along the back and neck.

‣ Increases flexibility of the spine and improves posture.

‣ Helps to open the flow of Qi along the "thoracic gate" on the mid-back and the "Jade pillow gate" on the upper neck area.

Chapter 9

Daoist Yoga Exercises for the Small Intestine Energy Meridian

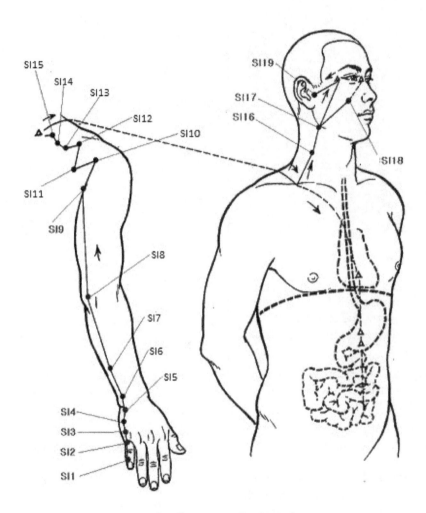

Small intestine Qi channel

Pathway of the Qi channel

The small intestine channel starts from the lateral side of the little finger. It ascends along the lateral aspect of the hand and reaches the little finger side of the wrist. It then travels up the posterior medial aspect of the forearm, crosses the elbow joint between the two bones, and follows the upper arm to the posterior aspect of the shoulder. The channel continues over the shoulder blade area, the back of the shoulder, and the posterior aspect of the neck. It then runs up moving posterior to the corner of the jaw bone and further up into the face to the cheeks before ending in front of the ear. This channel has 19 vital points.

Internal branches

1. From the top of the shoulder a branch runs over the collar bone, moves into the chest, and connects to the heart. It then follows down through the diaphragm, along the stomach, and links to the small intestine.

2. A second branch comes out from the shoulder region and runs up the neck to the cheek. It travels to the outer corner of the eye and then enters the ear.

3. A branch detaches from the small intestine and descends to the anterior aspect of the lower leg (Stomach 39).

4. Another branch separates from the main channel at the jaw, rises to the area below the eye, and ends at the inner corner of the eye.

Main signs of imbalance

Signs of excess (Fullness of Qi)

Abdominal pain, pain in the lower abdomen that may radiate down to the testicles or the lower back, abdominal bloating, rumbling of the intestines, blood or mucus in the stool, pain on the lateral aspect of the shoulder and arm, pain at the lateral aspect of the elbow, pain in the armpit that extends to the shoulder blade and neck, stiffness of the neck, pain in the cheeks, tearing of the eye, pain in the ear, and small warts.

Signs of weakness (Emptiness of Qi)

Diarrhea, lower abdominal distention, rumbling of the intestines, loose stools, poor appetite, poor assimilation of nutrients, loss of weight, poor tone and weakness of the muscles along the course of the small intestine channel.

Main areas covered

Small finger, lateral wrist, posterior medial aspect of forearm, elbow and upper arm, posterior aspect of shoulder, shoulder blade area, posterior aspect of neck, area below jaw, cheeks, ear, eyes, heart, stomach, small intestine, and lateral aspect of lower leg.

CARRYING THE TRAY

Main vital points

Small Intestine 1 (lesser marsh) on the lateral side of the little finger, Small Intestine 3 (back ravine) proximal to the joint of the knuckle of the small finger, Small Intestine 4 (Yang pool) on the lateral side of the hand between the base of the 5th metacarpal bone and the wrist bone, Conception Vessel 10 (lower stomach) two inches above the navel, Small Intestine 9, 10 and 11 located on the shoulder blade area, Governing Vessel 20 (hundred meeting) at the top of the head.

Main muscle groups

Biceps brachii (anterior aspect of upper arm), supinator (lateral superior aspect of forearm), **anterior deltoid** (anterior aspect of shoulder between lateral collar bone and upper arm), **pectoralis major** (chest region from chest bone and medial collar bone to upper arm), flexor carpi ulnaris (posterior medial aspect of forearm, between lateral elbow and base of fifth finger), extensor carpi ulnaris (posterior aspect of forearm between lateral aspect of elbow and base of fifth finger), posterior deltoid (posterior aspect of shoulder between shoulder blade and upper arm), **triceps** (posterior aspect of upper arm between upper arm and elbow), **latissimus dorsi** (from crest of hip bone, sacrum, and lower thoracic vertebrae across middle and lower back to posterior aspect of upper arm), teres minor (lateral inferior aspect of shoulder blade), **teres major** (from inferior angle of shoulder blade to medial aspect of upper arm), infraspinatus (shoulder blade region), subscapularis (anterior aspect of shoulder blade), supraspinatus (superior aspect of shoulder blade).

Secondary muscle groups

Serratus anterior (chest wall between upper 8 ribs and anterior surface of shoulder blade), pectoralis minor (chest region between anterior 3, 4, and 5 ribs and anterior shoulder blade).

Starting position

Step forward with the left foot into a left forward bow stance with the feet shoulder-width apart.

Description of the exercise

1 Place the right hand on the hip and extend the left hand with palm up in front of the abdomen.

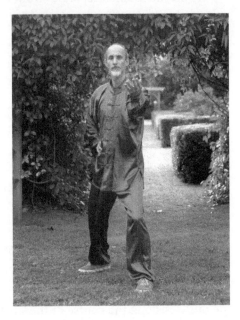

CARRYING THE TRAY

2 Rotate the left hand medially toward the mid-abdomen, shifting the weight to the right leg.

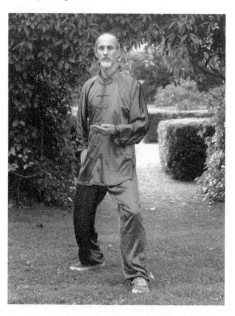

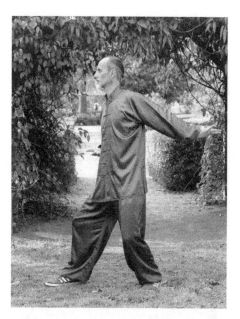

3 In a continuous movement turn the wrist medially in the direction of the little finger, moving the left hand along the ribs, and then extend the arm back with the palm facing up as breathing in.

4 Rotate the left hand medially and to the front with the palm still facing up, at the same time shifting the weight to the left leg and breathing out.

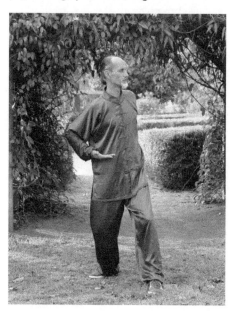

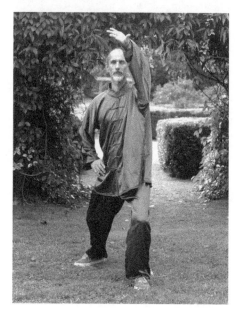

CARRYING THE TRAY

5 Continue rotating the left hand medially and then bending the elbow move the hand back over the head with palm facing up.

At the same time shift the weight to the right leg as breathing in. The dorsum of the left hand should be facing the top of the head.

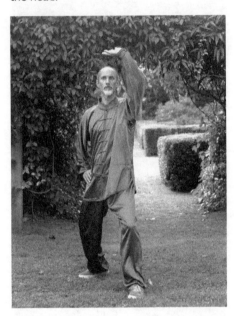

6 In a continuous motion rotate the left hand out and then to the front, again shifting the weight to the left leg and breathing out. Keep the left palm facing up and focus the mind on the little finger side of the hand.

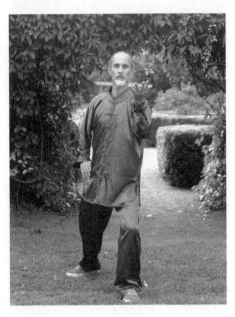

7 Bring the left hand in toward the mid-abdomen, shifting the weight to the right leg while breathing in.

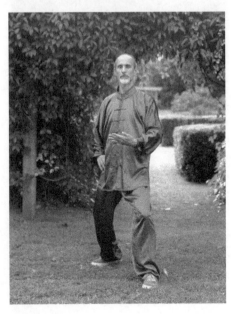

CARRYING THE TRAY

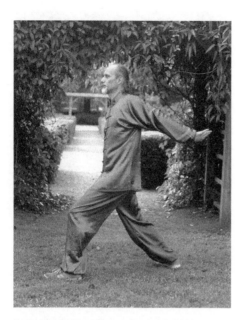

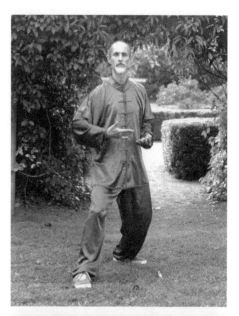

8 Repeat the exercise several times.

9 Step back with the left foot and repeat the exercise with the right foot in front.

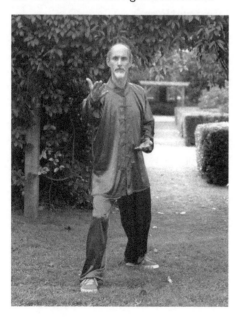

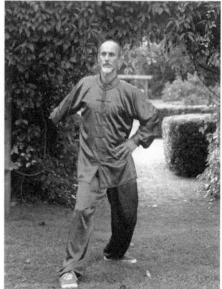

CARRYING THE TRAY

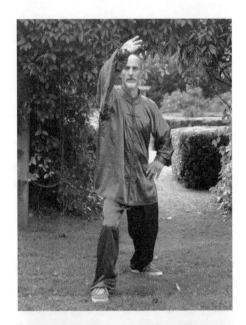

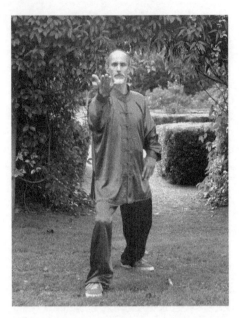

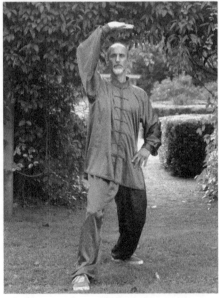

10 End the exercise by stepping back with the right foot and bringing the hands to the lower *Dantian*.

Observations

‣ Make sure to keep the palm facing up throughout the exercise as if you were carrying a tray.

‣ Maintain the shoulders lowered and wrist relaxed.

Breathing method

Generally during this exercise breathe in when moving the hand medially and toward the body. Breathe out when moving the hand out and toward the front of the body.

CARRYING THE TRAY

Flow of Qi

Qi flows from the mid-abdomen up the shoulder blade area and out from the lateral aspect of the arm and hand along the small intestine Qi channel.

Mind focus

Focus on maintaining the palm up throughout the exercise as if carrying a tray, as well as on the little finger side of the arm and hand, keeping the shoulders lowered, and coordinating the movements with the breathing.

Main Qi channel

Small intestine.

Secondary Qi channel

Heart.

Main benefits

› Increases flexibility of the shoulders, shoulder blades, arms, and neck along the pathway of the small intestine channel.

› Relieves stiffness of the neck and pain of the lateral aspect of the shoulder and arm.

› Helps relieve signs of abdominal bloating, lower abdominal pain, rumbling of the intestines, loose stools, and constipation.

› Promotes the flow of Qi or vital energy along the small intestine channel.

SWIMMING ON AIR

Main vital points

Small Intestine 1 (lesser marsh) on the lateral side of the small finger proximal to the corner of the nail, Small Intestine 3 (back ravine) on the lateral side of the hand proximal to the knuckle of the fifth finger, Small Intestine 4 (Yang pool) on the lateral side of the hand between the base of the fifth metacarpal bone and the wrist bone, Small Intestine 9 (true shoulder) one inch above the posterior crease of the armpit, Small Intestine 10 (upper arm *Shu*) and Small Intestine 11 (celestial gathering) on the shoulder blade area, Large Intestine 15 (shoulder bone) on the lateral anterior aspect of the shoulder joint.

Main muscle groups

Pronator teres (anterior aspect of forearm across from medial elbow to middle of lateral radius bone), pronator quadratus (horizontally across wrist on anterior aspect), **posterior deltoid** (posterior aspect of shoulder between shoulder blade and upper arm), pectoralis major (chest region from chest bone and medial collar bone to upper arm), **middle trapezius** (upper back area from thoracic vertebrae to spine of shoulder blade), **rhomboids** (shoulder blade area from thoracic vertebrae to medial border of shoulder blade), **infraspinatus** (shoulder blade region), **teres minor** (lateral inferior aspect of shoulder blade), serratus anterior (chest wall between upper 8 ribs and anterior surface of shoulder blade), splenius capitis (from spinous processes of C7, T1, T2, and T3 to mastoid bone and occipital bone).

Secondary muscle groups

Flexor carpi ulnaris (posterior medial aspect of forearm, between lateral elbow and base of fifth finger), anterior deltoid (anterior aspect of shoulder between lateral collar bone and upper arm), middle deltoid (lateral superior aspect of upper arm), pectoralis minor (chest region between anterior 3, 4, and 5 ribs and anterior shoulder blade), teres major (from inferior angle of shoulder blade to medial aspect of upper arm).

Starting position

Stand with the feet shoulder-width apart and hands by the sides.

Description of the exercise

1 Raise the arms in front of the chest with the elbows bent and palms facing down.

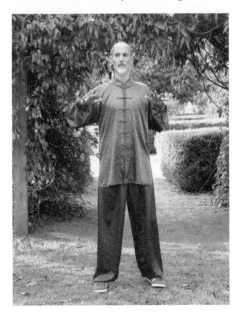

SWIMMING ON AIR

2 Move the hands to the front of the body while breathing out.

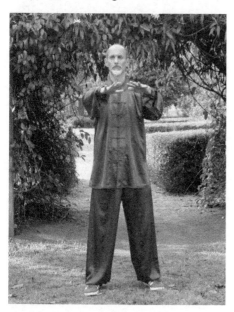

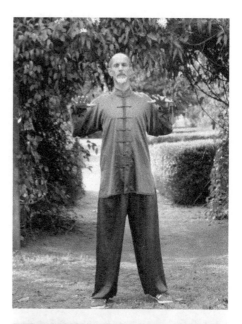

3 In a continuous motion rotate the hands out and then back, squeezing the shoulder blades while breathing in.

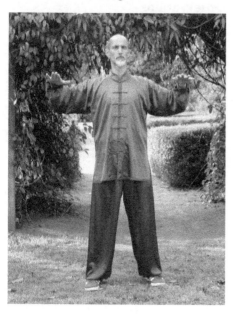

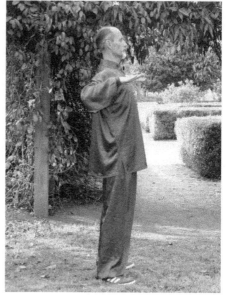

SWIMMING ON AIR

4 Repeat the movement several times.

5 Move the hands down the front of the body, rotating the palms up and bringing the lateral side of the small finger (Small Intestine 1) in contact with the Conception Vessel 10 point two inches above the navel. At the same time lower the head, bow the back and bend the knees.

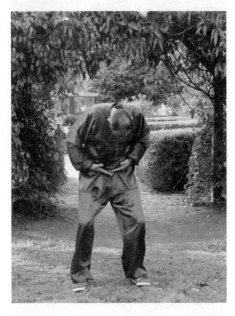

6 Slowly raise the head up and back, stretching and opening the chest and rib cage areas as breathing in.

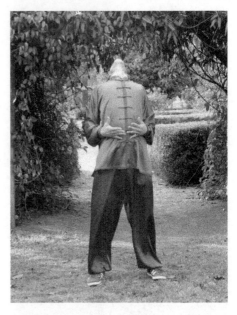

7 Repeat the head and chest stretch two times more.

8 End the exercise by bringing the hands to the lower *Dantian*.

Observations

‣ Keep the palms flat and facing down throughout the exercise.

‣ Maintain the shoulders lowered.

‣ Move the arms on a flat or horizontal plane.

Breathing method

Breathe out when moving the hands forward, when lowering the hands to the abdomen and when straightening the head. Breathe in when rotating the hands back and when stretching the head back.

SWIMMING ON AIR

Flow of Qi

Qi flows from the chest out to the hands and back to the shoulder blades area along the small intestine Qi channel.

Mind focus

Focus on moving the hands along a flat plane as if you were touching a flat smooth surface, squeezing and flattening the shoulder blades, relaxing the hands, keeping the shoulders lowered, and the flow of Qi along the small intestine channel.

Main Qi channel

Small intestine.

Secondary Qi channels

Heart, conception vessel (*Ren Mai*).

Main benefits

‣ Opens the shoulder blade area, activating the small intestine Qi channel.

‣ Relieves tightness of the shoulders, shoulder blades, upper back, and neck areas.

‣ Activates the flow of Qi through the upper back, shoulders, arm, and hands.

Chapter 10

Daoist Yoga Exercises for the Urinary Bladder Energy Meridian

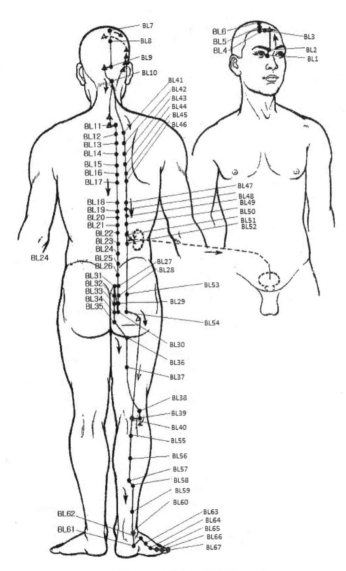

Urinary bladder Qi channel

Pathway of the Qi channel

The urinary bladder channel starts at the inner corner of the eye, moves up the forehead, and travels over the head to the back of the neck. It then runs down along the back two fingers lateral to the posterior midline of the body to the sacrum bone area. The channel continues out from the buttocks and down the posterior aspect of the thigh, posterior knee, and the posterior lower leg to the lateral ankle bone. It follows along the lateral side of the foot and ends at the lateral side of the little toe. This is the longest Qi channel of the body with 67 vital points along its pathway.

Internal branches

1. From the Urinary Bladder 7 point on top of the head a branch runs to the vertex of the head and enters the brain. From the vertex a branch goes down the sides of the head to the area above the ears.

2. From the lower back a branch travels to the kidneys and connects with the urinary bladder.

3. From the buttocks a branch connects to the Gall Bladder 30 point on the hip joint.

Main signs of imbalance

Signs of excess (Fullness of Qi)

Chills, fever, pain and tearing of the eyes, dizziness, yellow discoloration of the eyes, nasal congestion, frontal sinusitis, occipital headache, tightness, pain and stiffness of the neck, mania, epilepsy, stiffness of the back muscles, pain along the back, lower back pain, generalized spasm along the back (opisthotonos), sensation of coldness and pain along the Qi channel, lower abdominal pain and distention, difficult and painful urination, cramping and spasm of the hamstring and calf muscles, and pain and paralysis of the legs.

Signs of weakness (Emptiness of Qi)

Chronic clear nasal discharge, some cases of nosebleed, urinary incontinence, sensation of lower abdominal distention, weak and dribbling urination, hemorrhoids, and prolapse of the bladder.

Main areas covered

Inner corner of eye, forehead, top of head, brain, neck, along back, buttocks, hamstrings, posterior aspect of knee, calf, lateral ankle, lateral heel, lateral side of foot, little toe, urinary bladder, and kidneys.

GREETING THE IMMORTALS

Main vital points

Small Intestine 3 (back gorge) proximal to the knuckle of the little finger, Urinary Bladder 23 (kidney transport) on the lower back region two fingers lateral to the second lumbar vertebra, Urinary Bladder 28 (urinary bladder transport) on the sacrum lateral to the second sacral hole, Urinary Bladder 62 (extending vessel) in the depression inferior to the tip of the lateral ankle bone, Urinary Bladder 1 (bright eyes) 0.1 inches superior to the inner corner of the eye, Governing Vessel 23 (upper star) on the midpoint of the forehead one inch within the anterior hairline, Governing Vessel 20 (hundred meetings) on the vertex of the head, Urinary Bladder 16 (governing transport) two fingers lateral to the sixth thoracic vertebra, Urinary Bladder 15 (heart transport) two fingers lateral to the fifth thoracic vertebra, Urinary Bladder 14 (extreme Yin transport) two fingers lateral to the fourth thoracic vertebra, Urinary Bladder 44 (spirit hall) three inches lateral to the fifth thoracic vertebra, Urinary Bladder 43 (*Gao Huang* transport) three inches lateral to the fourth thoracic vertebra.

Main muscle groups

Upper trapezius (neck and shoulder region between neck vertebrae and lateral aspect of collar bone), anterior deltoid (anterior aspect of shoulder between lateral collar bone and upper arm), pectoralis major (chest region from chest bone and medial collar bone to upper arm), **erector spinae** (along back between vertebrae, posterior ribs, and occipital bone), **multifidus** (along spine from transverse processes of vertebrae to spinous processes spanning 2 to 4 vertebral segments), rectus abdominis (anterior aspect of abdomen between pubic bone and lower end of chest bone), **hamstrings** (posterior upper leg from sitting bone to posterior aspect of knee), tibialis anterior (anterior aspect of lower leg on shin bone), **peroneous longus** (lateral aspect of lower leg), **peroneous brevis** (lateral lower leg from lower half of tibia bone to base of fifth toe), quadratum lumborum (lower back area from posterior hip bone to lumbar vertebrae and 12th rib).

Secondary muscle groups

Pectoralis minor (chest region between anterior 3, 4, and 5 ribs and anterior shoulder blade), teres minor (lateral inferior aspect of shoulder blade), teres major (from inferior angle of shoulder blade to medial aspect of upper arm), **popliteus** (posterior aspect of knee), splenius capitis (from spinous processes of C7, T1, T2, and T3 to mastoid bone and occipital bone), splenius cervicis (from upper thoracic vertebrae of T3–T6 to upper cervical vertebrae of C1, C2, and C3).

Starting position

Stand with the feet together and hands by the sides.

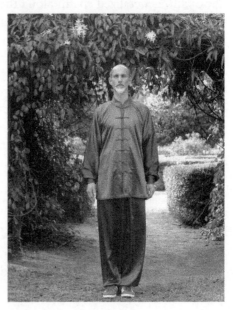

GREETING THE IMMORTALS

Description of the exercise

1 Cross the right arm over the left, bringing the back of the hands together.

2 Stretch both arms straight up over the head, following the arms with the eyes while breathing in.

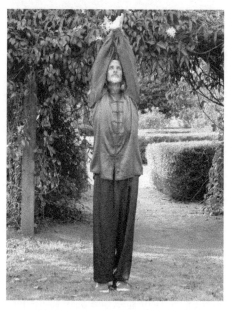

3 Bend the body down from the hips until the hands reach the floor between the feet as breathing out.

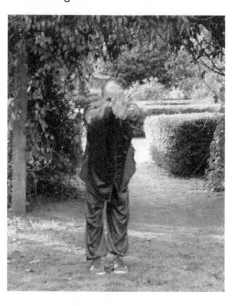

4 Turn the body to the left and bring the crossed hands to the side of the left ankle while breathing in.

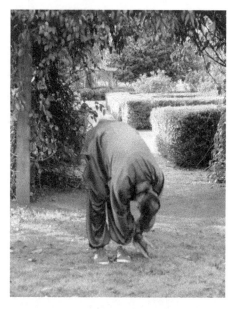

5 Bring the body back to the center between the two feet as breathing out.

6 Turn the body to the right and bring the hands to the side of the right ankle as breathing in.

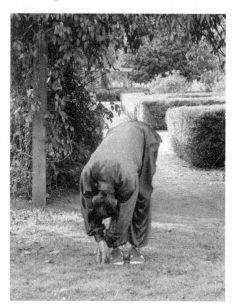

GREETING THE IMMORTALS

7 Bring the hands back to the center while breathing out.

8 Slowly straighten up the body, stretching the arms all the way above the head. Keep the arms crossed and the back of the hands held together. At the same time follow the movement of the arms with the eyes while breathing in.

9 Bend the elbows and bring the hands down over the head with palms up. Rest the dorsum of the right hand over the front of the head and the left hand on top of the right. At the same time breathe out.

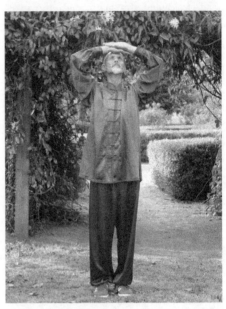

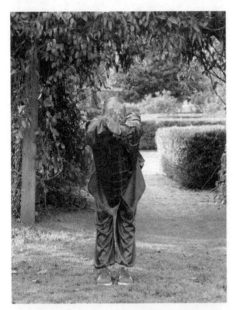

10 First bend the body to the left side, then to the right side, and back to the left side again. Breathe in with the body in the neutral position and breathe out when bending the body to the sides.

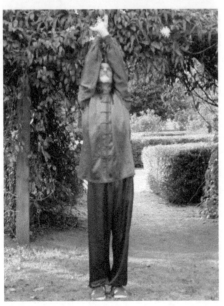

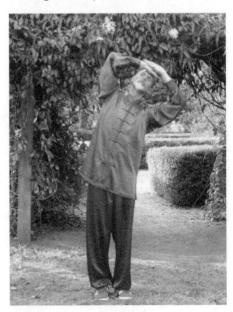

GREETING THE IMMORTALS

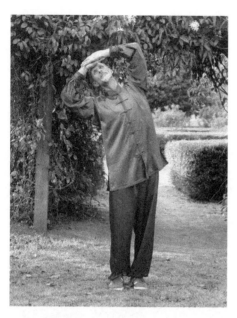

11 Stretch the hands up over the head, crossing the left arm over the right with the back of the hands held together. At the same time breathe in.

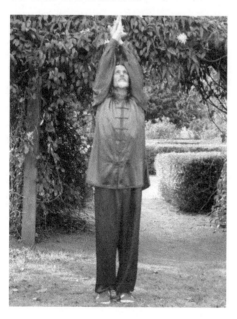

12 Bend the body down from the hips until the hands reach the floor between the feet while breathing out.

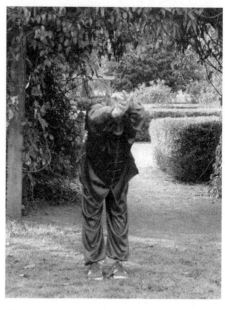

13 Repeat the movement this time first turning the body to the side of the right ankle and then to the side of the left ankle.

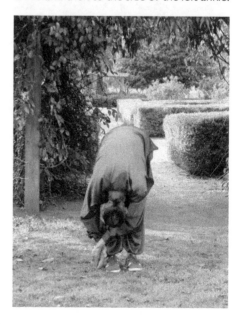

GREETING THE IMMORTALS

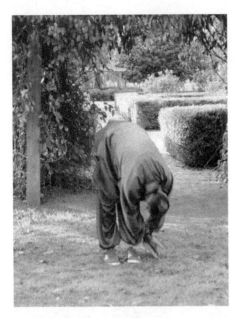

14 Straighten up the body, stretching the hands all the way above the head, breathing in. Keep the back of the hands together.

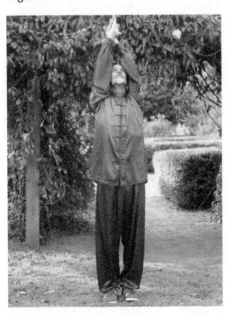

15 Lower the hands down the sides, breathing out.

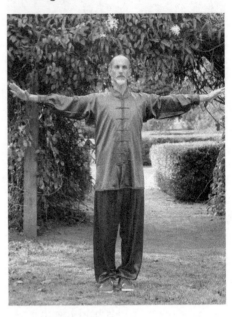

Observations

‣ Bend the body down from the hips and not the back.

‣ When bending the body down, hold the hips stable.

‣ Keep the arms straight and aligned with the ears when bending down and straightening the body.

‣ Coordinate the movements with the breathing.

GREETING THE IMMORTALS

Precautions and contraindications

This exercise can be contraindicated in cases of slipped or herniated lumbar disc, sciatica, serious back conditions, high blood pressure, heart disease, and vertigo.

Breathing method

Breathe in when raising the arms, when turning the body down to the sides, and when straightening up the body. Breathe out when lowering the body and when bending the body sideways.

Flow of Qi

Qi flows up the back to the top of the head (Governing Vessel 20) and the arms, then down the back and the posterior aspect of the legs along the urinary bladder Qi channel to the sides of the heels.

Mind focus

Focus on bending from the hips, keeping the arms aligned with the ears and the back straight, and the flow of Qi along the urinary bladder Qi channel.

Main Qi channels

Urinary bladder, Yang motility vessel (*Yang Qiao Mai*).

Secondary Qi channels

Governing vessel (*Du Mai*), small intestine, kidney.

Main benefits

‣ Stretches the back and the posterior leg muscles along the urinary bladder Qi channel.

‣ Helps to relieve stiffness and pain of the lower back, waist, and hips.

‣ Improves flexibility of the spine.

‣ Relieves tightness of the upper back, shoulders, and lower back.

‣ Activates the Yang motility channel (*Yang Qiao Mai*), thus promoting the flow of vital energy along the legs, back, shoulders, neck, head, and eyes.

‣ Stimulates the flow of Qi or vital energy along the urinary bladder channel.

‣ Stimulates and strengthens the kidneys.

BENDING THE WAIST AND TURNING THE SACRUM

Main vital points

Small Intestine 3 (back gorge) proximal to the knuckle of the little finger, Urinary Bladder 1 (bright eyes) 0.1 inches superior to the inner corner of the eye, Urinary Bladder 2 (bamboo gathering) on the medial corner of the eyebrow, Governing Vessel 23 (upper star) on the midpoint of the forehead one inch within the anterior hairline, Governing Vessel 20 (hundred meetings) on the vertex of the head, Urinary Bladder 23 (kidney transport) on the lower back region two fingers lateral to the second lumbar vertebra, Urinary Bladder 28 (urinary bladder transport) on the sacrum lateral to the second sacral hole, Urinary Bladder 30 (white ring *Shu*) on the sacrum lateral to the fourth sacral bone, Urinary Bladder 32 (second bone hole) on the second sacral hole, Urinary Bladder 35 (meeting of Yang) half an inch lateral to the tip of the coccyx, Urinary Bladder 40 (bend middle) posterior to the knee, Urinary Bladder 57 (mountain support) on the calf eight inches below the midpoint of the knee.

Main muscle groups

Biceps brachii (anterior aspect of upper arm), anterior deltoid (anterior aspect of shoulder between lateral collar bone and upper arm), **rectus abdominus** (abdomen area from pubic bone to inferior aspect of breast bone), erector spinae (along back between vertebrae, posterior ribs, and occipital bone), **biceps femoris** (posterior aspect of upper leg from sitting bone to lateral aspect of knee), **semimembranosus** (posterior upper leg from sitting bone to posterior knee), **semitendinosus** (posterior upper leg from sitting bone to posterior knee), transverse abdominis (horizontally across abdomen from back to front), **internal oblique** (lateral aspect of abdomen from anterior hip bone to lower 4 ribs and abdomen), **external oblique** (lateral abdomen from lower 8 ribs to abdomen and hip bone), **sternocleidomastoid** (anterior lateral aspect of neck from superior chest bone and medial collar bone to mastoid bone behind ear), splenius capitis (from spinous processes of C7, T1, T2, and T3 to mastoid bone and occipital bone), splenius cervitis (from upper thoracic vertebrae of T3–T6 to transverse processes of upper cervical vertebrae of C1, C2, and C3).

Secondary muscle groups

Pectoralis minor (chest region between anterior 3, 4, and 5 ribs and anterior shoulder blade), pronator teres (anterior aspect of forearm across from medial elbow to middle of lateral radius bone), pronator quadratus (horizontally across proximal aspect of anterior wrist), flexor carpi ulnaris (posterior medial aspect of forearm, between lateral elbow and base of fifth finger), quadratus lumborum (lower back area between posterior hip bone and lumbar vertebrae), flexor digitorum superficialis (anterior aspect of forearm and hand), flexor digitorum profundus (anterior aspect of forearm, hand, and fingers).

Starting position

Stand with the feet together and hands by the sides.

BENDING THE WAIST AND
TURNING THE SACRUM

Description of the exercise

1 Bring the hands together with the palms of the hands facing, as if holding a vase in front of the lower abdomen.

2 Scoop the hands out and up in front of the body all the way over the head.

3 In a continuous motion rotate the hands in and down the body with the fingers pointing downward, quickly bending the body down from the hips. The hands make a loose fist in front of the lower legs.

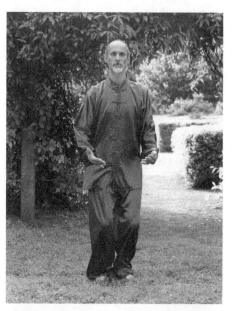

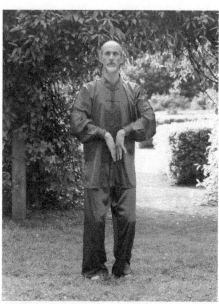

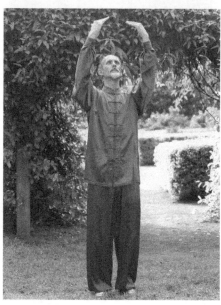

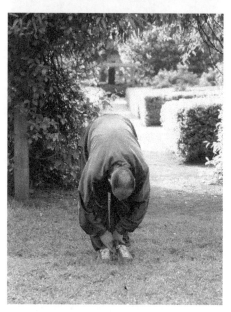

BENDING THE WAIST AND
TURNING THE SACRUM

4 In a continuous movement describe small forward circles with the fists down the front of the legs, the left leg, front of the legs, the right leg, and the front of the legs again. At the same time move the lower spine area up and down along with the fists.

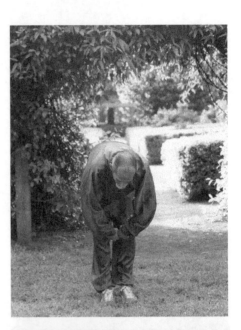

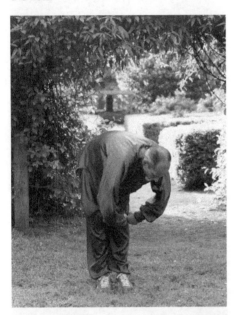

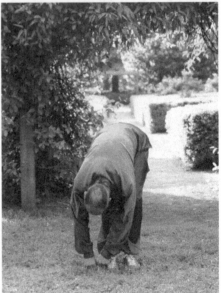

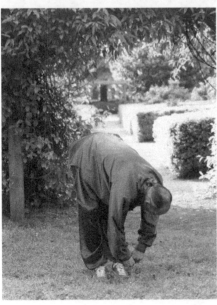

BENDING THE WAIST AND
TURNING THE SACRUM

5 Supporting the fists on the lower legs hold the hips back, lengthening the lower spine and lifting the head gazing up at the superior inner corner of the eyebrows (Urinary Bladder 1 and Urinary Bladder 2). This action activates the urinary bladder Qi channel.

6 Turn the hips to the right side at the same time turning the head to the left side and looking back. Then turn the hips to the left side at the same time turning the head to the right side and looking back. Alternate the movement turning the hips to the right and left sides several times.

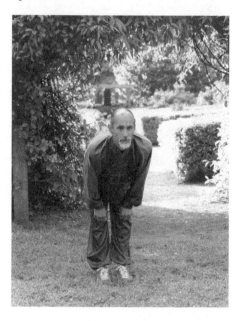

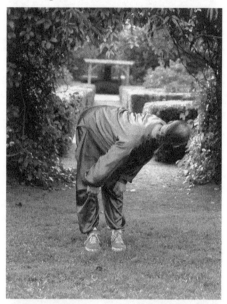

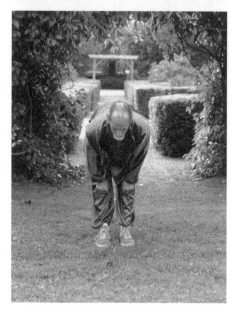

BENDING THE WAIST AND
TURNING THE SACRUM

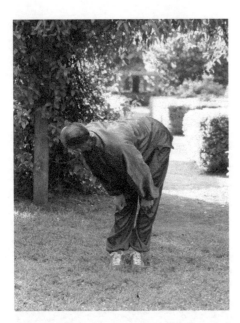

7 Scoop the hands out and up in front of the body and over the head.

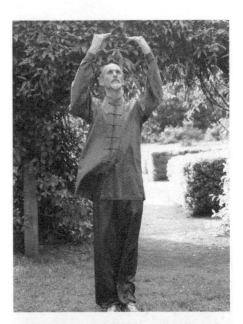

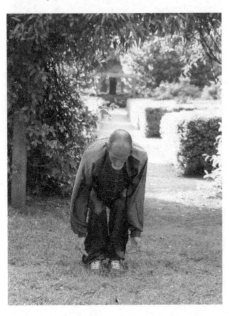

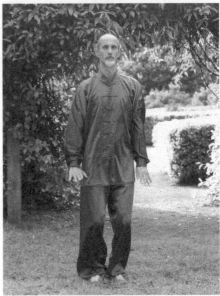

8 Scoop the hands in and down the front of the body to the lower *Dantian*.

9 Repeat the exercise three to four times.

BENDING THE WAIST AND TURNING THE SACRUM

Observations

‣ Hold the hips back when straightening the spine and turning the body to the sides.

‣ Be sure to move the lower spine up and down along with the movement of the fists.

‣ Turn the hips and head in opposite directions while lengthening the lower spine.

‣ When lifting the head, gaze up at the inner corner of the eyes.

Precautions and contraindications

This exercise may be contraindicated for people with acute lower back pain, bulging or herniated lumbar disc, high blood pressure, severe dizziness, hernia, and sciatic nerve pain.

Breathing method

Breathe in when scooping the hands up, when circling the fists up the front of the legs, and when raising the body. Breathe out when bending the body, when circling the fists down the front of the legs, and when lowering the hands.

Flow of Qi

Qi flows up the front of the body to the top of the head (Governing Vessel 20) and down the back of the body and the posterior aspect of the legs along the urinary bladder Qi channel. When turning the lower spine Qi flows up and down the left and right sides of the back.

Mind focus

Focus on bending down from the hips, holding the head up, looking at the superior inner corner of the eyebrows, holding back the hips, and turning and stretching the lower spine.

Main Qi channel

Urinary bladder.

Secondary Qi channels

Large intestine, governing vessel (*Du Mai*), Yang motility vessel (*Yang Qiao Mai*).

Main benefits

‣ Stretches the lower spine and sacral area.

‣ Alternately stretches and compresses the left and right sides of the back.

‣ Helps to relieve stiffness and pain of the lower back.

‣ Activates the energy flow along the back.

‣ Helps to open the tailbone gate and lengthen the lower end of the spine.

‣ Stimulates the parasympathetic nerves along the neck and lower spine, thus calming and refreshing the nervous system.

Chapter 11

Daoist Yoga Exercises for the Kidney Energy Meridian

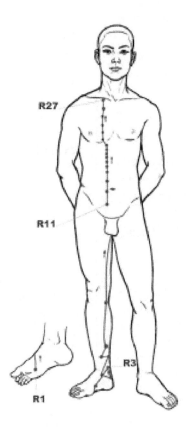

Kidney Qi channel

Pathway of the Qi channel

The kidney channel starts from the sole of the foot and it moves up over the arch of the foot to the inner ankle area. It then travels up the posterior medial aspect of the lower leg, the posterior aspect of the knee, and further up along the posterior medial aspect of the thigh. The channel ascends to the pubic region half an inch from the anterior midline of the body and continues up the lower and the upper abdomen. Moving out to the ribs the channel runs up the chest to end below the collar bone two inches lateral to the anterior midline of the body. The kidney channel has 27 vital points.

Internal branches

1. From the point Urinary Bladder 67 on the little toe an internal branch runs out over the sole of the foot to the point Kidney 1.

2. From the upper thigh the channel enters the base of the spine at the point Governing Vessel 1, continues up the spine to the lower back where it moves to the kidneys, and then connects to the urinary bladder in the lower abdomen.

3. From the kidneys a branch ascends to the liver, goes through the diaphragm, enters the lungs, runs along the throat, and ends at the back (root) of the tongue.

4. Another branch comes out from the lungs, connects to the heart, and disperses in the chest to link with the pericardium channel.

Main signs of imbalance

Signs of excess (Fullness of Qi)

Pain in the posterior inner aspect of the leg, cramping, spasm, twisting or pain along the course of the kidney channel, chronic vaginal discharge abundant in amount (leucorrhea), difficult urination or bowel movement, sensation of heaviness and tightness of the lower back.

Signs of weakness (Emptiness of Qi)

Weakness and soreness of the lower back and waist area, lack of tone of the lower back muscles, coldness of the lumbar region, lower back pain, coldness of the lower extremities, weakness of the legs and knees, water retention or edema, swollen ankles, knees, or legs, grey, dark, and dull facial complexion, depression, mild dizziness, ringing in the ears of long standing and low pitch (tinnitus), hearing loss, loss of memory, impotence, frigidity, low sex drive, premature ejaculation, infertility, menstrual disorders, delayed onset of the first menstrual period (menarche), scanty menstruation or absence of menses (amenorrhea), history of miscarriages, frequent urination, incontinence of urine, weak or dribbling urination, chronic diarrhea, and shortness of breath with difficulty on inhalation.

Main areas covered

Bottom of foot, medial ankle, inner heel, posterior medial aspect of lower leg, knee and thigh, lower abdomen, middle abdomen, ribs, chest, area inferior to collar bone, lower spine, kidneys, bladder, lower back, liver, lungs, heart, posterior throat, and root of tongue.

STRENGTHENING THE KIDNEY
AND GUIDING QI

Main vital points

Large Intestine 4 (joined valleys) on the dorsum of the hand between the thumb and first finger, Kidney 27 (*Shu* mansion) below the collar bone two inches from the midline, Urinary Bladder 23 (kidney transport) on the lower back 1.5 inches from the second lumbar vertebra, Governing Vessel 4 (life gate) on the lower back between the second and third lumbar vertebra, Urinary Bladder 44 (spirit hall) three inches lateral from the fifth thoracic vertebra, Gall Bladder 26 (girdle vessel) on the side of the waist in line with the navel and inferior to the eleventh rib, Large Intestine 15 (shoulder bone) on the upper arm lateral anterior to the shoulder joint.

Main muscle groups

Gluteus maximus (on buttocks from sacrum to thigh bone), iliopsoas (core muscles between lumbar vertebrae and head of thigh bone), **posterior deltoid** (posterior aspect of shoulder between shoulder blade and upper arm), biceps brachii (anterior aspect of upper arm), infraspinatus (shoulder blade region), rhomboids (shoulder blade area from thoracic vertebrae to medial border of shoulder blade), **quadratus lumborum** (lower back area between posterior hip bone and lumbar vertebrae), **external oblique** (lateral aspect of abdomen from lower 8 ribs to abdomen and hip), **internal oblique** (lateral aspect of abdomen from anterior hip bone to lower 4 ribs and abdomen), sternocleidomastoid (anterior lateral aspect of neck from superior chest bone and medial collar bone to mastoid bone behind ear), splenius capitis (from spinous processes of C7, T1, T2, and T3 to mastoid bone and occipital bone), splenius cervitis (posterior aspect of neck from upper thoracic vertebrae to upper cervical vertebrae), **multifidus** (along back from transverse processes of vertebrae to spinous processes spanning 2 to 4 vertebral segments), **rotators** (on back from transverse processes of vertebrae to spinous processes of vertebrae directly above).

Secondary muscle groups

Upper trapezius (neck and shoulder region between neck vertebrae and lateral aspect of collar bone), middle trapezius (upper back area from thoracic vertebrae to spine of shoulder blade), pectoralis major (chest region from chest bone and medial collar bone to upper arm), teres minor (lateral inferior aspect of shoulder blade), rectus femoris (anterior aspect of thigh between pelvis and kneecap).

Starting position

Stand with the feet slightly wider than the hips.

STRENGTHENING THE KIDNEY
AND GUIDING QI

Description of the exercise

1 Bend the knees, at the same time relaxing the hips and straightening the lower back.

2 Place the dorsum of the hands over the lower back area. Make sure to keep the shoulders lowered and the lower back area lengthened and relaxed. In this position breathe in while focusing on the lower back area and breathe out while focusing on the kidneys for seven times.

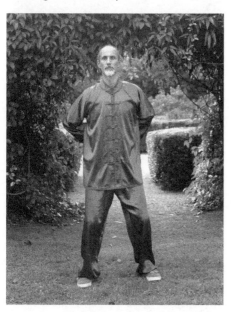

3 Turn the body from the waist to the left side, looking over the shoulder to the back as you breathe out.

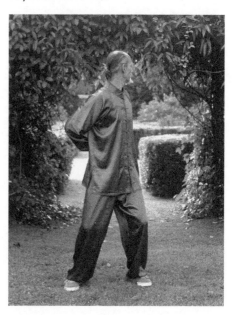

4 Turn the body back to the center while breathing in.

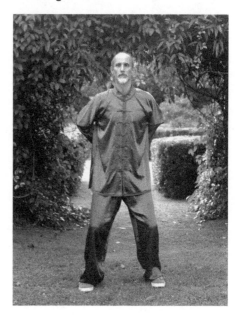

STRENGTHENING THE KIDNEY
AND GUIDING QI

5 Turn the body from the waist to the right side, looking over the shoulder to the back as you breathe out.

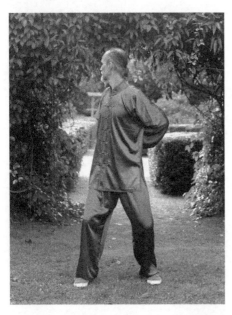

6 Return the body to the center position while breathing in.

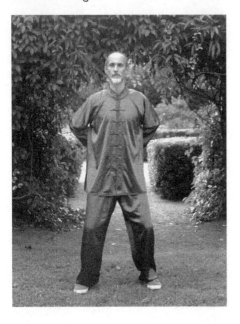

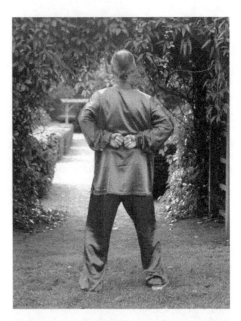

7 Continue turning to the left and right sides for several times.

8 End the exercise by bringing the hands to the lower *Dantian*.

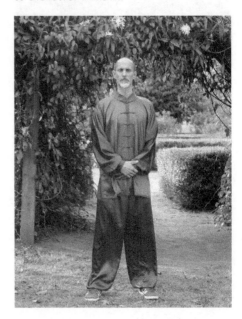

STRENGTHENING THE KIDNEY AND GUIDING QI

Observations

- Make sure the lower back area is not arched, but slightly rounded.

- Turn from the waist and not the shoulders.

- Coordinate the turning of the body with the breathing.

- Keep the shoulders lowered.

Precautions and contraindications

Do not practice this exercise if having a cold, fever, congestion, or an acute infectious disease.

Breathing method

Breathe in with the body in the center position. Breathe out when turning the body to the sides.

Flow of Qi

Qi flows from the dorsum of the hands (Large Intestine 4) to the lower back and the kidneys (Urinary Bladder 23). When turning the body to the sides Qi flows into the waist area and the right and left sides of the back.

Mind focus

Keeping the lower back rounded, relaxing the waist, turning from the waist, and the flow of Qi between the left and right sides of the lower back.

Main Qi channels

Kidney, urinary bladder.

Secondary Qi channels

Gall bladder, three heaters, large intestine.

Main benefits

- Strengthens the kidney Qi and promotes kidney functions.

- Helps to relieve signs of weak kidney Qi including impotence, premature ejaculation, menstrual disorders, frequent urination, urine incontinence, infertility, menopausal symptoms, depression, tinnitus, and cold limbs.

- Relaxes the waist and back areas.

- Relieves tightness, soreness, and pain of the lower back.

- Energizes the life gate fire (*Ming Men*), increasing overall vitality.

- Stimulates the production of *Jing* (essence) and hormonal secretions.

- Helps to balance the hormones and strengthen the reproductive system.

SCOOPING THE MOON FROM THE WATER

Main vital points

Pericardium 8 (labored palace) on the center of the palms between the second and third metacarpal bones, Kidney 1 (gushing spring) on the bottom of the foot, Kidney 27 (*Shu* mansion) below the collar bone two inches from the midline, Conception Vessel 4 (origin pass) four fingers below the navel, Urinary Bladder 23 (kidney transport) on the lower back 1.5 inches from the second lumbar vertebra, Gall Bladder 30 (jumping round) in the buttock region on the hip joint.

Main muscle groups

Biceps brachii (anterior aspect of upper arm), **upper trapezius** (neck and shoulder region between neck vertebrae and lateral aspect of collar bone), **teres minor** (lateral inferior aspect of shoulder blade), teres major (from inferior angle of shoulder blade to medial aspect of upper arm), serratus anterior (chest wall between upper 8 ribs and anterior surface of shoulder blade), anterior deltoid (anterior aspect of shoulder between lateral collar bone and upper arm), gluteus maximus (buttock area from hip bone to lateral aspect of thigh), **rectus femoris** (anterior aspect of thigh between pelvis and kneecap), pectineus (inner thigh from pubic bone to upper thigh bone), adductor longus and adductor brevis (inner thigh from pubic bone to posterior thigh bone), iliopsoas (core muscles between lumbar vertebrae and head of thigh bone), popliteus (posterior aspect of knee), posterior deltoid (posterior aspect of shoulder between shoulder blade and upper arm), supinator (lateral superior aspect of forearm).

Secondary muscle groups

Pectoralis major (chest region from chest bone and medial collar bone to upper arm), tibialis anterior (anterior aspect of lower leg on shin bone).

Starting position

Stand with the feet slightly wider than the hips, knees slightly flexed and hands by the sides.

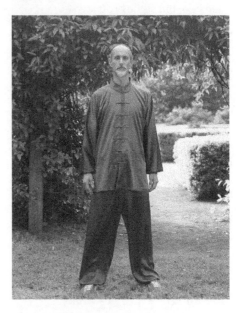

Description of the exercise

1 Bending from the waist, move the hands down along the lateral aspect of the legs to the midpoint between the feet as you breathe out.

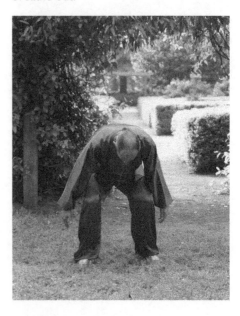

SCOOPING THE MOON FROM THE WATER

2 Turn the palms up with the fingers of both hands facing, as if lifting a heavy object from the ground. At the same time bend the knees, squatting down.

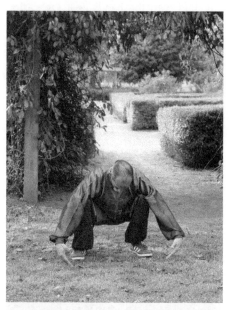

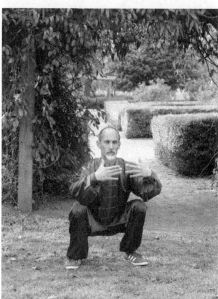

3 Slowly straighten the body, bringing the hands up the front until the hands reach the chest level as you breathe in. End with the hands in the position of embracing a balloon with the palms facing the body.

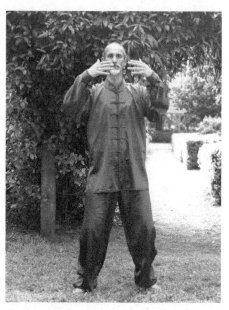

4 Move the hands in and down the front of the body to the lower abdominal area as you breathe out.

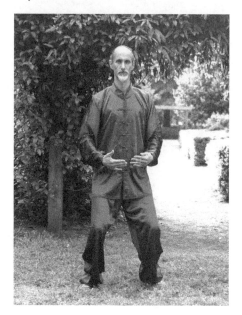

SCOOPING THE MOON FROM THE WATER

5 Continue moving the hands toward the back along the hips and up to the kidneys with the palms of the hands facing the body as you breathe in.

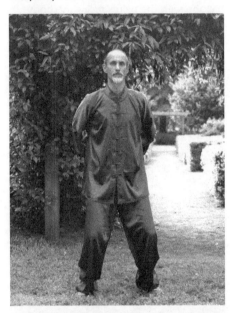

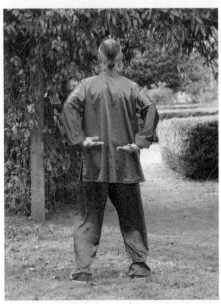

6 In a continuous movement bring the hands up the back as you breathe in, then under the armpits and around the ribs to the front of the chest as you breathe out. End with the hands as if embracing a balloon.

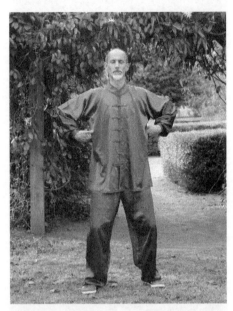

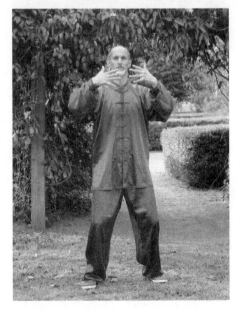

SCOOPING THE MOON FROM THE WATER

7 Move the hands down to the lower abdomen as you breathe in.

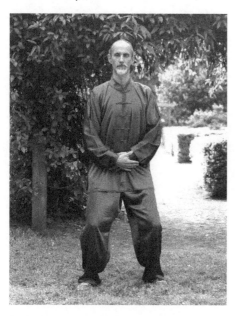

8 Repeat the exercise six times.

9 End the exercise by bringing the hands to the lower *Dantian*.

Observations

‣ When lifting the hands from the ground, visualize holding a bright-white round object like the full moon, and guiding the flow of Qi up the medial aspect of the legs to the lower *Dantian* center.

‣ When squatting down, try to maintain the body as straight as possible.

‣ Squat down only as far as comfortable. If full squatting is not possible, lift the heels when bending the knees.

‣ When bringing the hands down to the midpoint between the feet, keep the knees slightly bent.

Precautions and contraindications

This exercise may be contraindicated in cases of serious back conditions, sciatica, high blood pressure, heart disease, and vertigo.

Breathing method

Breathe out when bending the body down and when lowering the hands. Breathe in when lifting the hands and when moving the hands up the back.

Flow of Qi

First, Qi flows down the legs to the bottom of the feet (Kidney 1). It then flows up the legs along the kidney Qi channel to the chest (Kidney 27), down the front of the body to the *Dantian*, up the back to the kidneys, further up along the urinary bladder Qi channel on the back, and down to the lower *Dantian*.

Mind focus

Guiding the Qi down when bending the body then up when straightening the body, maintaining the lower back and hips relaxed, and coordinating the movements of the body with the breathing.

Main Qi channels

Kidney, urinary bladder.

Secondary Qi channels

Spleen, liver, stomach, gall bladder.

Main benefits

‣ Strengthens the legs and core muscles.

‣ Activates the flow of Qi or vital energy in the pelvis, lower back, and legs.

‣ Strengthens the kidney and the original Qi of the body (prenatal Qi).

‣ Helps gather Yin Qi from the earth and supports women's health in cases of infertility, menstrual imbalances, menopausal symptoms, and reproductive disorders.

‣ Stimulates the flow of Qi along the kidney, liver, spleen, urinary bladder, gall bladder, and stomach channels.

Chapter 12

Daoist Yoga Exercises for the Pericardium Energy Meridian

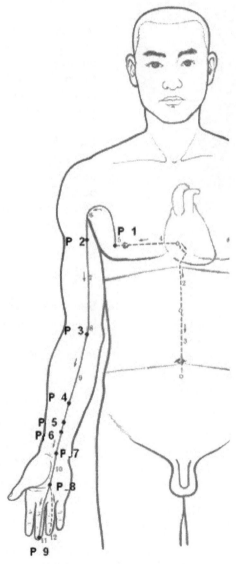

Pericardium Qi channel

Pathway of the Qi channel

The pericardium channel starts inside the chest, travels laterally across the chest and comes out to the surface of the body one inch lateral to the nipple at the ribs region. The channel moves up along the anterior aspect of the armpit to the upper arm. It then runs down the anterior midline of the upper arm, the elbow crease medial to the biceps tendon, and further down the lower arm between the two main tendons to the midpoint of the wrist. It continues down the center of the palm between the second and third fingers to end at the tip of the middle finger. This channel has nine vital points.

Internal branches

1. From the chest a branch runs down through the diaphragm into the abdomen to connect to the upper, middle, and lower heaters.

2. Another branch comes out from the palm (Pericardium 8) and runs to the lateral aspect of the ring finger (Three Heaters 1).

Main signs of imbalance

Signs of excess (Fullness of Qi)

Fullness and pain of the lateral rib region, swelling of the area below the armpit, spasm of the arm, contraction and tightness of the elbow and arm restricting movement, hot palms, pain on the medial aspect of the elbow and arm, heart pain, fullness and oppression of the chest, palpitations, vomiting, stomach pain, nausea, epilepsy, mania and depression, incoherent speech, mental disorders, certain feverish diseases (e.g. malaria), flushed face, and loss of consciousness.

Signs of weakness (Emptiness of Qi)

Cold hands, poor tone, weakness and flaccidity of the muscle along the course of the channel, feeling of uneasiness in the heart and chest area, restlessness, palpitations with sensation of emptiness, susceptibility to fright, and poor blood circulation.

Main areas covered

Pericardium, chest, armpit, rib region, anterior midline of upper arm, elbow and forearm, palm, middle finger, upper abdomen, and lower abdomen.

TWO ELBOWS REELING

Main vital points

Pericardium 6 (inner pass) two inches above the anterior midpoint of the wrist, Pericardium 8 (labored palace) on the center of the palm between the second and third metacarpal bones, Pericardium 3 (marsh at the bend) on the center of the elbow crease medial to the biceps tendon, Conception Vessel 17 (middle of the breasts) on the center of the chest, Conception Vessel 4 (origin pass) four fingers below the navel.

Main muscle groups

Gluteus maximus (buttock area from hip bone to lateral aspect of thigh), adductor longus (upper inner thigh from pubic bone to posterior aspect of thigh bone), **posterior deltoid** (posterior aspect of shoulder between shoulder blade and upper arm), teres minor (lateral inferior aspect of shoulder blade), **serratus anterior** (chest wall between upper 8 ribs and anterior surface of shoulder blade), **upper trapezius** (neck and shoulder region between neck vertebrae and lateral aspect of collar bone), lower trapezius (middle back between thoracic vertebrae and root of spine of shoulder blade), **pectoralis minor** (chest region between anterior 3, 4, and 5 ribs and anterior shoulder blade), **anterior deltoid** (anterior aspect of shoulder between lateral collar bone and upper arm), **rhomboid** (shoulder blade from upper thoracic vertebrae to medial border of shoulder blade), levator scapulae (shoulder blade region from upper neck vertebrae to superior aspect of shoulder blade), biceps brachii (anterior aspect of upper arm), **brachialis** (anterior inferior aspect of upper arm between upper arm bone and ulna bone).

Secondary muscle groups

Teres major (from inferior angle of shoulder blade to medial aspect of upper arm), latissimus dorsi (from crest of hip bone, sacrum, and lower thoracic vertebrae across middle and lower back to posterior aspect of upper arm), infraspinatus (shoulder blade region), subscapularis (anterior aspect of shoulder blade), pectoralis major (chest region from chest bone and medial collar bone to upper arm), **pronator teres** (anterior aspect of forearm across from medial elbow to middle of lateral radius bone), **flexor carpi radialis** (anterior aspect of forearm, between lateral elbow and bases of second and third fingers), **palmaris longus** (anterior aspect of forearm from medial humerus bone to palm of hand), flexor pollicis brevis (anterior aspect of hand from wrist bones to base of thumb), flexor digiti minimi (anterior aspect of hand from wrist to base of proximal phalanx of little finger), lumbricals (palm aspect of hand), flexor digitorum superficialis (anterior aspect of forearm and hand), **flexor digitorum profundus** (anterior aspect of forearm, hand, and fingers), flexor pollici longus (anterior aspect of forearm from middle of radial bone to distal phalanx of thumb).

TWO ELBOWS REELING

Starting position

Stand in a horse-riding stance with the feet about twice the width of the shoulders.

Description of the exercise

1 Cross the forearms about two inches above the wrists with loose fists.

2 Bend the knees and lower the body into a middle-height horse-riding stance.

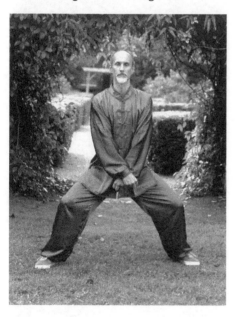

3 Bring the arms up along the trunk, rotating the elbows up to chest level while straightening the knees. In a continuous movement rotate the elbows out moving the fists to the sides while keeping contact with the body.

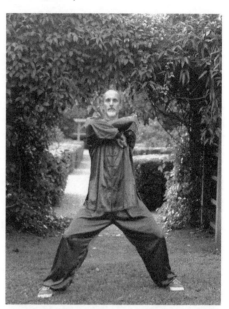

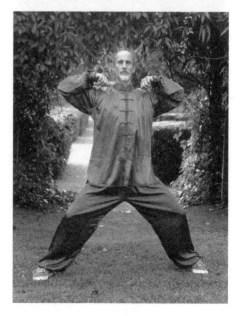

TWO ELBOWS REELING

4 Continue rotating the elbows then extend the arms out and down the sides of the body with elbows slightly bent until the fists cross again in front of the lower abdomen. At the same time bend the knees lowering the body.

5 Repeat the movement several times.

6 Reverse the direction of the movement, raising the fists along the sides of the trunk and rotating the elbows up the sides of the body to chest level.

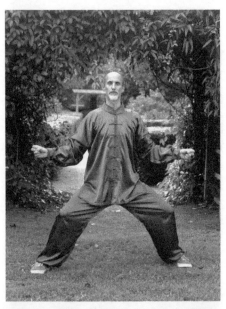

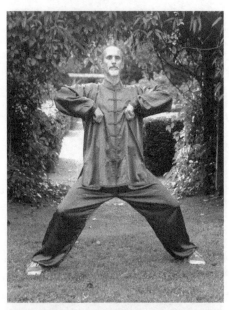

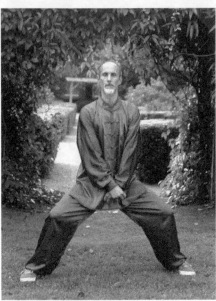

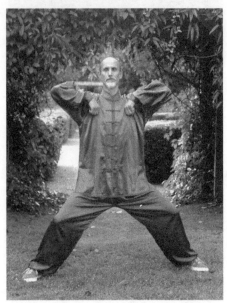

TWO ELBOWS REELING

7 In a continuous motion rotate the elbows forward, then crossing and extending the arms in front of the chest and down the front of the body to the *Dantian*. At the same time bend the knees lowering the body.

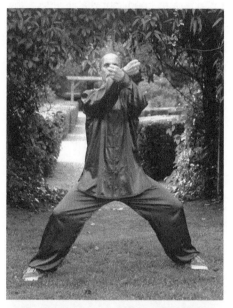

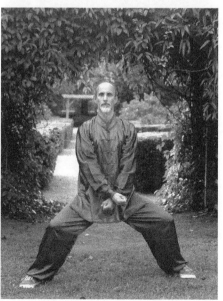

8 Repeat the movement several times.

9 End the exercise by bringing the hands to the lower *Dantian*.

Observations

‣ When moving the hands up the front and when moving the hands up the sides, keep the fists in contact with the body.

‣ When rotating the elbows up open the chest breathing in, and when rotating the elbows down close the chest breathing out.

‣ Raise and lower the body in coordination with the movements of the arms.

Breathing method

Breathe in when rotating the elbows up and raising the body. Breathe out when rotating the elbows down and lowering the body.

Flow of Qi

Qi flows up the trunk and the ribs to the chest region, then out from the arms along the Pericardium Qi channel and down the trunk to the lower *Dantian*.

Mind focus

Focus on rotating the elbows and fists, opening and closing the chest, and coordinating the movements of the body with the breathing.

Main Qi channels

Pericardium, Yin linking vessel (*Yin Wei Mai*).

Secondary Qi channels

Three heaters, conception vessel (*Ren Mai*), thrusting vessel (*Chong Mai*), gall bladder, liver.

TWO ELBOWS REELING

Main benefits

‣ Relieves tightness and pressure of the diaphragm muscle and the chest region.

‣ Works out the chest, shoulders, and upper back.

‣ Stimulates heart and lung function.

‣ Increases flexibility of the shoulders and elbows.

‣ Activates the flow of original Qi (*Yuan Qi*) between the lower *Dantian* (lower abdomen) and the middle *Dantian* (chest region), improving general health.

‣ Strengthens the legs and the core muscles.

‣ Stimulates important vital points on the wrists, arms, and elbows that benefit the heart, calm the mind, settle the stomach, and relieve chest and rib pain.

‣ Strengthens the kidneys.

PUSHING DOWN THE TIGER

Main vital points

Pericardium 6 (inner pass) two inches above the anterior midpoint of the wrist, Pericardium 8 (labored palace) on the center of the palm between the second and third metacarpal bones, Conception Vessel 17 (middle of the breasts) on the center of the chest, Conception Vessel 4 (origin pass) four fingers below the navel, Spleen 4 (yellow emperor) on the medial side of the foot distal to the base of the first metatarsal bone.

Main muscle groups

Biceps brachii (anterior aspect of upper arm), **brachialis** (anterior inferior aspect of upper arm between upper arm bone and ulna bone), supinator (lateral superior aspect of forearm), rhomboids (shoulder blade area from thoracic vertebrae to medial border of shoulder blade), **pectoralis major clavicular head** (from medial half of collar bone to upper arm), **pronator teres** (anterior aspect of forearm across from medial elbow to middle of lateral radius bone), **pronator quadratus** (horizontally across anterior aspect of wrist), **gluteus maximus** (buttock area from hip bone to lateral aspect of thigh), adductor longus (upper inner thigh from pubic bone to posterior aspect of thigh bone), middle deltoid (lateral superior aspect of upper arm), supraspinatus (superior aspect of shoulder blade), middle trapezius (upper back area from thoracic vertebrae to spine of shoulder blade), extensor carpi radialis longus (posterior aspect of forearm between lateral aspect of elbow and base of second finger), extensor carpi radialis brevis (posterior aspect of forearm between lateral aspect of elbow and base of third finger).

Secondary muscle groups

Triceps (posterior aspect of upper arm between upper arm and elbow), biceps femoris (posterior aspect of upper leg from sitting bone to lateral aspect of knee), gastrocnemius (calf muscle on posterior aspect of lower leg between knee and heel bone), soleus (posterior aspect of lower leg), popliteus (posterior aspect of knee), extensor hallucis longus (anterior aspect of lower leg from anterior fibula bone to distal joint of big toe), extensor digitorum brevis (anterior aspect of foot from ankle bone to four medial toes), extensor digitorum longus (anterior aspect of lower leg from fibula and tibia bones to four lateral toes).

Starting position

Stand in a middle-height horse-riding stance with the feet wider than the shoulders and the hands facing up in front of the lower abdomen.

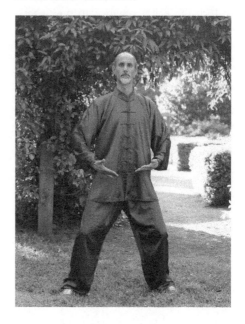

PUSHING DOWN THE TIGER

Description of the exercise

1 Raise the body moving the hands up to chest level as you breathe in.

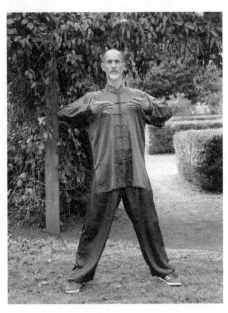

2 Turn the palms down with the fingers of both hands facing each other, and then quickly drop the body, pushing down with the palms as you breathe out.

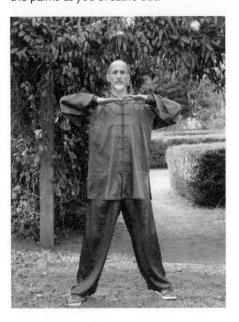

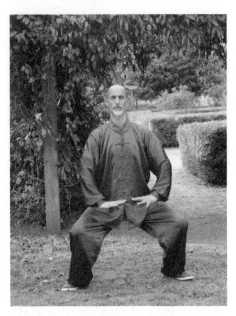

3 Turn the palms up and repeat the movement several times.

4 End the exercise by bringing the hands to the lower *Dantian*.

Observations

‣ When dropping the body down, raise the heels off the floor, focusing the action of the movement on the point Spleen 4 on the arch of the feet.

‣ Keep the body upright throughout the exercise.

‣ When pushing down with the palms, flex the wrists to stimulate the points Pericardium 6 and Pericardium 8 located near the wrists and on the palms.

‣ Maintain the fingertips of the hands facing each other.

PUSHING DOWN THE TIGER

Breathing method

Breathe in when moving the hands up to chest level and raising the body. Breathe out when pushing the hands down and lowering the body.

Flow of Qi

Qi flows up and down between the lower *Dantian* and the chest, and down the legs along the spleen Qi channel.

Mind focus

Focus on the action of pushing and dropping down with the body, the flow of Qi between the lower *Dantian* and the chest area, and coordinating the movements of the body with the breathing.

Main Qi channel

Pericardium.

Secondary Qi channels

Three heaters, conception vessel (*Ren Mai*), spleen, Yin linking vessel (*Yin Wei Mai*).

Main benefits

‣ Circulates Qi or vital energy between the kidneys (water) and the heart (fire), thus promoting overall energy balance.

‣ Helps link the flow of Yin Qi from the legs up into the trunk and compressing Yang Qi down into the lower *Dantian*.

‣ Strengthens the tendons, muscles, and joints.

‣ Stimulates blood flow and oxygen delivery to the tissues.

‣ Activates the Yin linking channel (*Yin Wei Mai*). This vessel is in charge of linking the flow of Yin Qi in the body and strengthening the balance of energy between the interior and the surface of the body.

‣ Supports the liver Qi and strengthens the kidneys.

‣ Relieves tightness of the chest, stomach pain, vomiting, and acid reflux.

Chapter 13

Daoist Yoga Exercises for the Three Heaters Energy Meridian

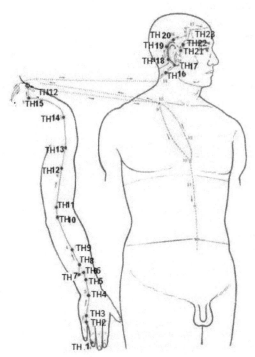

Three heaters Qi channel

Pathway of the Qi channel

The three heaters channel starts from the lateral side of the ring finger and runs along the dorsum of the hand between the ring and little finger to the midpoint of the wrist. It travels upward along the posterior midline of the forearm between the radius and the ulna bones, runs through the elbow, and then moves up the upper arm to the posterior lateral aspect of the shoulder. The channel continues running posterior to the shoulder and up the lateral aspect of the neck to the area behind the ear. It then travels up behind and around the ear to the temple area, ending at the lateral side of the eyebrow. This channel has 23 vital points along its pathway.

Internal branches

1. From the point Three Heaters 15 behind the shoulder a branch moves over the shoulder and the collar bone into the chest to connect with the pericardium. It continues down through the diaphragm, middle abdomen, and lower abdomen connecting the three heaters.

2. From the chest a branch runs upward to the neck, curves behind the ear and follows further up along the anterior hairline to the corner of the forehead. It then moves down in front of the ear to the cheek region and ends in the area below the eye.

3. From the point Three Heaters 17 on the area behind the ear a branch enters the ear. It then comes out in front of the ear and crosses the cheek area to the lateral corner of the eye (Gall Bladder 1) where it connects with the gall bladder channel.

4. From the lower abdomen another branch moves down the posterior aspect of the leg to the posterior knee area (Urinary Bladder 39).

Main signs of imbalance

Signs of excess (Fullness of Qi)

Temporal headache, redness of the eyes, ringing in the ears (tinnitus), hearing loss, pain in the cheeks, pain behind the ears, fever, sore throat, malaria, sudden hoarseness of voice, neck pain, pain in the rib side region (hypochondriac region), pain, tension, and cramps on the posterior aspect of the shoulder, elbow, and arm along the course of the channel, tremor of the hand, curling of the tongue, bloating and fullness of the abdomen, sensation of hardness in the lower abdomen, and difficult urination.

Signs of weakness (Emptiness of Qi)

Lack of tone and weakness of the muscles around the elbow, frequent urination, water retention or edema, sensation of emptiness in the body, susceptibility to fright, and poor blood circulation.

Main areas covered

Ring finger, dorsum of hand, lateral aspect of arm, shoulder, and neck, ear, temples, lateral aspect of eyebrow and eye, corner of forehead, cheek region, area inferior to eyes, chest region, middle and lower abdomen, and posterior lateral aspect of knee.

THE EXERCISE OF THE THREE HEATERS

Main vital points

Conception Vessel 4 (origin pass) four fingers below the navel, Pericardium 8 (labored palace) on the palm of the hand between the second and third metacarpal bones, Conception Vessel 12 (middle stomach) four inches above the navel, Conception Vessel 17 (middle of the breasts) on the center of the chest, *Tian Mu* (heavenly eye) at the midpoint between the eyebrows, Governing Vessel 20 (hundred meeting) on top of the head.

Main muscle groups

Biceps brachii (anterior aspect of upper arm), brachialis (anterior inferior aspect of upper arm between upper arm bone and ulna bone), supinator (lateral superior aspect of forearm), pronator teres (anterior aspect of forearm across from medial elbow to middle of lateral radius bone), pronator quadratus (horizontally across anterior aspect of wrist), supraspinatus (superior aspect of shoulder blade), **teres minor** (lateral inferior aspect of shoulder blade), infraspinatus (shoulder blade region), gastrocnemius (calf muscle on posterior aspect of lower leg between knee and heel bone), soleus (posterior aspect of lower leg), anterior deltoid (anterior aspect of shoulder between lateral collar bone and upper arm), extensor carpi radialis (posterior aspect of forearm from lateral aspect of elbow to base of second and third fingers), extensor carpi ulnaris (posterior aspect of forearm between lateral aspect of elbow and base of fifth finger), extensor hallucis longus (anterior aspect of lower leg from anterior fibula bone to distal joint of big toe), extensor digitorum brevis (anterior aspect of foot from ankle bone to four medial toes), extensor digitorum longus (anterior aspect of lower leg from fibula and tibia bones to four lateral toes).

Secondary muscle groups

Posterior deltoid (posterior aspect of shoulder between shoulder blade and upper arm), middle deltoid (lateral superior aspect of upper arm), triceps brachii (posterior aspect of upper arm between upper arm and elbow), rhomboids (shoulder blade area from thoracic vertebrae to medial border of shoulder blade), plantaris (posterior aspect of lower leg).

Starting position

Stand with the feet shoulder-width apart, knees slightly flexed and hands by the sides.

Description of the exercise

1 Place the hands level with the lower abdomen with fingers facing each other and the palms up.

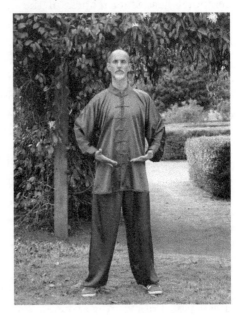

THE EXERCISE OF THE THREE HEATERS

2 Move the hands up to the chest level, at the same time raising the heels and breathing in.

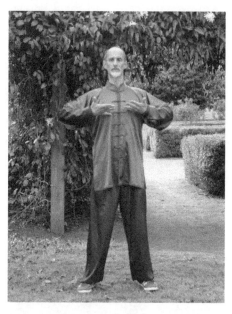

3 Turn the palms to face down and bring the hands down to the lower abdomen with fingers facing each other. At the same time drop the heels and breathe out.

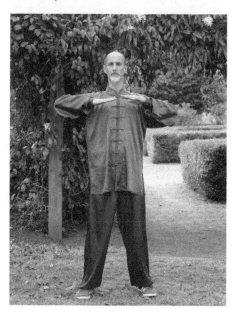

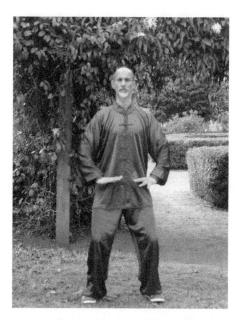

4 Repeat the movement several times.

5 Move the hands up to the chest level, raising the heels off the floor and breathing in. In a continuous movement rotate the palms out, moving the hands out and down the sides of the body with the palms facing down. At the same time drop the heels, bend the knees, and lower the body as you breathe out.

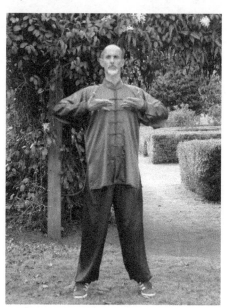

THE EXERCISE OF THE THREE HEATERS

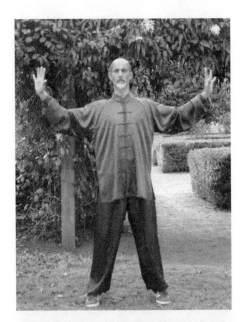

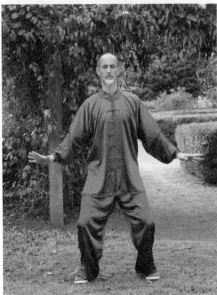

6 Bring the hands back to the lower abdomen with palms facing up and repeat the movement several times.

7 Move the hands up the midline of the body to the throat level, then rotate the hands out to face the front and extend them over the head with palms up and fingers facing. At the same time raise the heels as you breathe in.

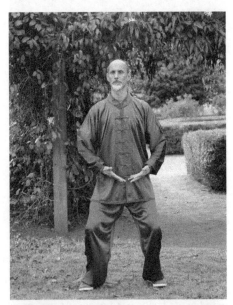

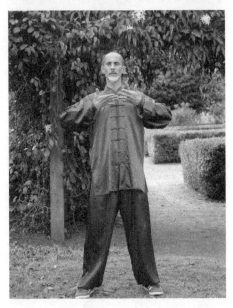

THE EXERCISE OF THE THREE HEATERS

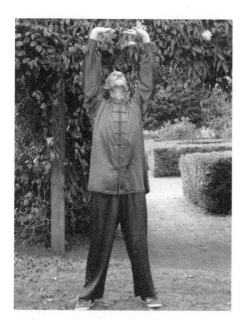

8 Move the hands out and down the sides of the body with the palms facing down. At the same time lower the heels and bend the knees as you breathe out.

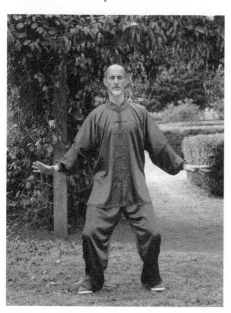

9 Repeat the movement several times.

10 At the end of the exercise bring the hands to the lower *Dantian*.

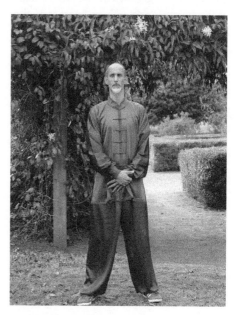

Observations

‣ Coordinate the movement of the hands, the raising and lowering of the body and heels, and the breathing.

‣ Keep the shoulders lowered and wrists soft throughout the exercise.

‣ When moving the hands up and down the front of the body keep the fingertips facing.

Breathing method

Breathe in when raising the hands. Breathe out when lowering the hands.

THE EXERCISE OF THE THREE HEATERS

Flow of Qi

Qi moves up and down the trunk and sides of the body along the three heaters of the body—the lower abdomen, the middle abdomen, and the chest and head—and also along the three heaters Qi channel.

Mind focus

Focus on the raising and lowering of the body, coordinating the movements with the breathing, and the flow of Qi up and down the body.

Main Qi channel

Three heaters.

Secondary Qi channels

Conception vessel (*Ren Mai*), lung, large intestine, stomach, pericardium, spleen.

Main benefits

‣ Promotes bowel movement, kidney function and elimination.

‣ Strengthens the digestive organs and improves digestive function.

‣ Stimulates breathing, blood circulation, and oxygenation of the tissues.

‣ Improves blood flow to the brain.

‣ Activates the system of endocrine glands and general metabolism.

‣ Stimulates fluid metabolism.

‣ Harmonizes the ascending and descending movement of Qi, thus enhancing energy exchange and transformation.

‣ Helps to balance the Yin and Yang energies of the body.

ACTIVATING THE THREE HEATERS

Main vital points

Triple Heater 4 (Yang pool) slightly lateral to the midpoint on the dorsum of the wrist, Conception Vessel 4 (origin pass) four fingers below the navel, Conception Vessel 12 (middle stomach) four inches above the navel, Conception Vessel 17 (middle of the breasts) on the center of the chest, *Tian Mu* (heavenly eye) on the midpoint between the eyebrows, Governing Vessel 20 (hundred meeting) on the top of the head.

Main muscle groups

Brachialis (lower half of anterior upper arm), **coracobrachialis** (anterior medial aspect of upper arm), **pectoralis minor** (chest region between anterior 3, 4, and 5 ribs and anterior shoulder blade), pronator teres (anterior aspect of forearm across from medial elbow to middle of lateral radius bone), **rhomboid** (shoulder blade region from upper thoracic vertebrae to medial border of shoulder blade), serratus anterior (chest wall between upper 8 ribs and anterior surface of shoulder blade), **infraspinatus** (shoulder blade region), **teres minor** (lateral inferior aspect of shoulder blade), **posterior deltoid** (posterior aspect of shoulder between shoulder blade and upper arm), levator scapulae (shoulder blade region from upper neck vertebrae to superior aspect of shoulder blade).

Secondary muscle groups

Scalenes (neck area from cervical vertebrae to first and second ribs), flexor carpi radialis (anterior aspect of forearm, between lateral elbow and bases of second and third fingers), flexor carpi ulnaris (posterior medial aspect of forearm, between lateral elbow and base of fifth finger), extensor carpi ulnaris (posterior aspect of forearm between lateral aspect of elbow and base of fifth finger), upper trapezius (neck and shoulder region between neck vertebrae and lateral aspect of collar bone), triceps (posterior aspect of upper arm between upper arm and elbow), pectoralis major (chest region from chest bone and medial collar bone to upper arm), latissimus dorsi (from crest of hip bone, sacrum, and lower thoracic vertebrae across middle and lower back to posterior aspect of upper arm).

Starting position

Stand with the feet wider apart than the shoulders and hands by the sides.

ACTIVATING THE THREE HEATERS

Description of the exercise

1 Shift the weight to the right leg and rotate the left foot 45 degrees out with the body turning over to the left.

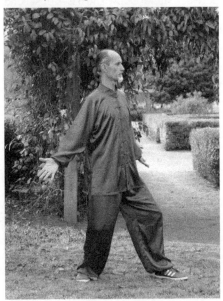

2 Shift the weight to the left leg, closing the front of the body from the chest down the upper and lower abdomen. At the same time round out the back and bring the dorsum of the hands together in front of the lower abdomen as you breathe in.

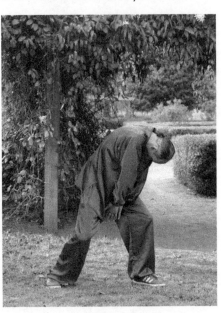

3 Move the hands up along the trunk opening the body from the lower abdomen to the upper abdomen and the chest and shifting the weight to the right leg. In a continuous movement quickly extend the hands up and out as you breathe out.

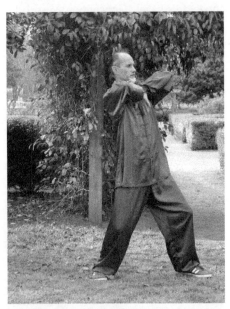

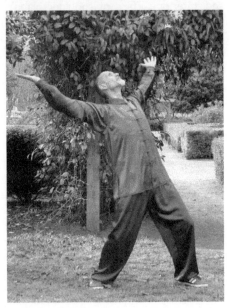

ACTIVATING THE THREE HEATERS

4 Rotate the hands out and down the sides, closing the front of the body from the chest down the upper and lower abdomen. At the same time shift the weight to the left leg rounding out the back, and bring the dorsum of the hands together in front of the lower abdomen as you breathe in.

5 Repeat the opening, closing, and opening movements of the trunk one time more.

6 After the last opening of the body shift the weight to the left leg and move the hands out and down the sides of the body hollowing the chest.

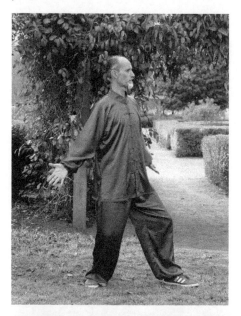

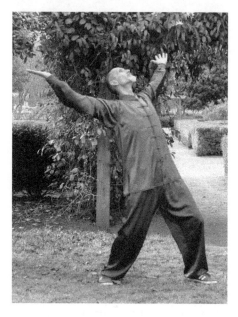

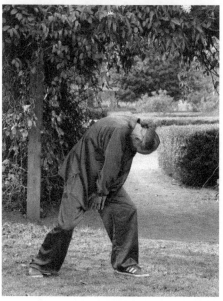

ACTIVATING THE THREE HEATERS

7 Keeping the weight on the left leg, turn the body to the right side rotating the right foot out 45 degrees and at the same time opening the chest and rotating the arms out.

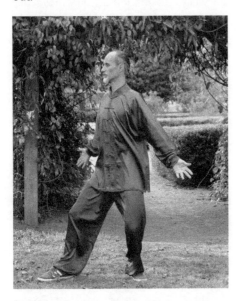

8 In a continuous motion close the front of the body from the chest down the upper and lower abdomen, shifting the weight to the right leg. At the same time bend the back and bring the dorsum of the hands together in front of the lower abdomen breathing in.

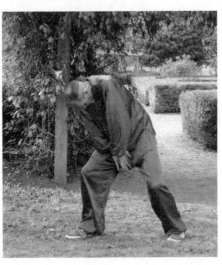

9 Move the hands up along the trunk opening the body from the lower abdomen to the upper abdomen and the chest, while shifting the weight to the left leg. In a continuous movement, quickly extend the hands up over the head as you breathe out.

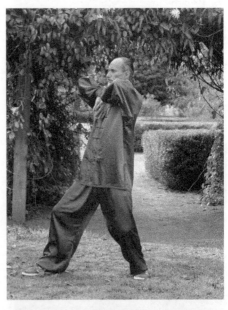

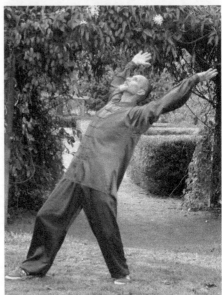

ACTIVATING THE THREE HEATERS

10 Rotate the hands out and down the sides, closing the front of the body from the chest down the upper and lower abdomen. At the same time shift the weight to the right leg and bring the back of the hands together in front of the lower abdomen as you breathe in.

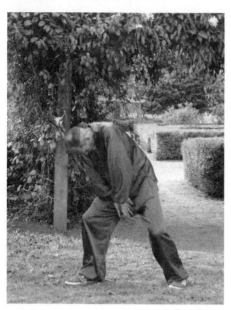

11 Repeat the opening, closing, and opening movements of the trunk one more time.

12 Alternate the exercise on the left and the right sides several times.

13 After the last opening movement of the trunk bring the hands over the head and down the front of the body to the lower *Dantian*.

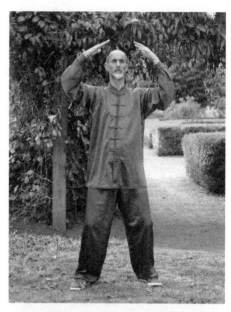

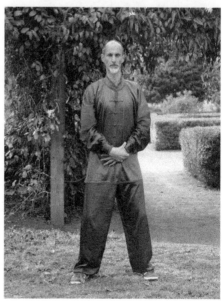

ACTIVATING THE THREE HEATERS

Observations

‣ Coordinate the movements of the body with the breathing.

‣ Alternate the opening and closing actions of the trunk and arms. The opening of the trunk takes place from the lower abdomen up to the chest, and the closing of the trunk takes place from the chest down to the lower abdomen.

Precautions and contraindications

This exercise may be contraindicated in cases of serious back conditions.

Breathing method

Breathe in when closing the trunk and arms. Breathe out when opening the trunk and arms.

Flow of Qi

Qi flows up the trunk along the three energy spaces of the body from the lower abdomen to the chest and head, and down from the head to the chest and lower abdomen. Qi also flows along the three heaters Qi channel along the arms.

Mind focus

Focus on opening and closing the trunk and arms, coordinating the movements with the breathing, and the flow of Qi along the three energy spaces of the body.

Main Qi channel

Three heaters.

Secondary Qi channels

Yang motility vessel (*Yang Qiao Mai*), conception vessel (*Ren Mai*), urinary bladder.

Main benefits

‣ Stimulates the opening and closing of the trunk.

‣ Activates energy flow along the trunk.

‣ Promotes the functions of digestion, elimination, and circulation.

‣ Improves flexibility of the spine and shoulders.

‣ Activates the three heaters Qi channel along the arms, shoulders, and neck.

Chapter 14

Daoist Yoga Exercises for the Gall Bladder Energy Meridian

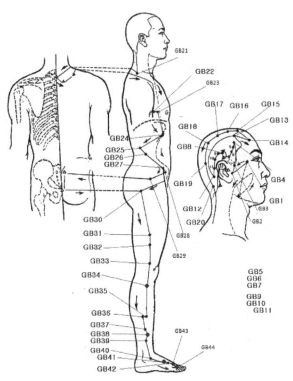

Gall bladder Qi channel

Pathway of the Qi channel

The gall bladder channel starts from the lateral corner of the eye, running out along the temples to the front of the ears, then up the side of the head to the corner of the forehead, and down the head around the posterior aspect of the ear to the mastoid bone behind the ear. It then moves medially up the side of the head to the forehead one inch above the midpoint of the eyebrows, and again curving up medially around the head to below the occipital bone. The channel continues down the side of the neck to the highest point of the shoulder and descends anterior to the armpit running down along the lateral ribs, the lateral waist, and the groin area where it moves out to the hip joint. The channel travels down the lateral midline of the thigh, the lateral aspect of the knee, and the lower leg to the anterior aspect of the lateral ankle bone. It then runs down over the dorsum of the foot between the fourth and fifth toes ending at the lateral side of the fourth toe. The gall bladder channel has 44 vital points.

Internal branches

1. From the lateral corner of the eye (Gall Bladder 1) a branch runs down to the jaw, up to the area below the eye, down the cheek, neck, and the area above the collar bone (Stomach 12) where it rejoins the main channel. It continues down over the shoulder to the chest, through the diaphragm, connects to the liver and enters the gall bladder. The internal branch runs down the ribs along the hypochondriac region coming out at the groin area, then goes around the genitals, and ends at the hip joint (Gall Bladder 30).

2. A branch separates from the main channel just above the collar bone at the shoulder (Stomach 12), runs down the armpit, and over the ribs region to below the eleventh rib (Liver 13) from where it travels over the back to the sacrum. From the sacrum the branch goes to the hip joint to reunite with the external channel.

3. A third branch comes out at the dorsum of the foot (Gall Bladder 41) and travels over the first and second metatarsal bones ending at the medial side of the big toe (Liver 1).

Main signs of imbalance

Signs of excess (Fullness of Qi)

Dizziness, temporal headache, migraine, pain and swelling of the eyes, stiffness and pain of the neck and shoulders, tinnitus, swollen nodes in the neck (scrofula), fullness and pain in the chest, swelling and pain in the armpit, pain in the hip and lateral aspect of the thigh and knee, hip joint pain, sciatica, alternation between chills and fever in acute diseases, bitter taste in the mouth, bilious vomiting, pain in the ribs and hypochondriac region, and jaundice.

Signs of weakness (Emptiness of Qi)

Deafness, dizziness, muscular atrophy with weakness and lack of tone of the lower limbs, difficulty standing with inability to walk, tendency toward constipation, difficulty digesting fats, difficulty making decisions, and timidity.

Main areas covered

Lateral eye, temples, area above eye, lateral head, ear, lateral neck, superior shoulder, anterior armpit, rib area, hypochondriac region, lateral waist, hip joint, lateral aspect of leg, lateral knee, lateral lower leg, anterior lateral ankle, and fourth toe.

BELT MERIDIAN GRINDING

Main vital points

Pericardium 8 (labored palace) on the palm between the second and third metacarpal bones, Gall Bladder 26 (girdle vessel) on the side of the waist in line with the navel and below the eleventh rib, Gall Bladder 24 (sun and moon) in line with the nipple between the seventh and eighth ribs, Gall Bladder 22 (armpit abyss) three inches below the center of the armpit, Gall Bladder 23 (sinew seat) one inch anterior to Gall Bladder 22, Stomach 25 (celestial pivot) two fingers lateral to the navel, Urinary Bladder 25 (large intestine transport) on the lower back 1.5 inches lateral to the fourth lumbar vertebra, Gall Bladder 21 on the highest point of the shoulder, Gall Bladder 30 (jumping round) on the buttock region at the hip joint.

Main muscle groups

Pectoralis minor (chest region between anterior 3, 4, and 5 ribs and anterior shoulder blade), serratus anterior (chest wall between upper 8 ribs and anterior surface of shoulder blade), posterior deltoid (posterior aspect of shoulder between shoulder blade and upper arm), **anterior deltoid** (anterior aspect of shoulder between lateral collar bone and upper arm), brachialis (anterior inferior aspect of upper arm between upper arm bone and ulna bone), pronator teres (anterior aspect of forearm across from medial elbow to middle of lateral radius bone), **external oblique** (lateral aspect of abdomen between lower 8 ribs and abdomen), **internal oblique** (lateral aspect of abdomen from anterior hip bone to lower 4 ribs and abdomen), transversospinalis (along back between transverse processes and spinous processes of vertebrae), rotators (from transverse processes to spinous processes of vertebrae).

Secondary muscle groups

Popliteus (posterior aspect of knee), pectoralis major (chest region from chest bone and medial collar bone to upper arm), rhomboid (shoulder blade area from upper thoracic vertebrae to medial border of shoulder blade), middle trapezius (upper back area from thoracic vertebrae to spine of shoulder blade), gluteus maximus (buttock area from hip bone to lateral aspect of thigh), **gluteus medius** (buttock area from crest of hip bone to head of thigh bone), **gluteus minimus** (buttock area from hip bone to anterior head of thigh bone), **peroneus tertius** (lateral aspect of lower leg from superior fibula bone to base of fifth toe).

Starting position

Stand with the feet wider than the hips, knees bent, and the palms facing down on the right side of the waist.

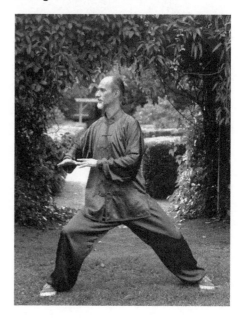

BELT MERIDIAN GRINDING

Description of the exercise

1 Turning from the waist, rotate the hands out to the left side, describing a small horizontal circle toward the left ribs. At the same time shift the weight to the left leg as you breathe in.

2 In a continuous movement rotate the hands in toward the left ribs, then turning from the waist rotate the hands back to the right side. At the same time shift the weight to the right leg as you breathe out.

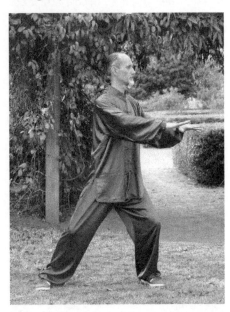

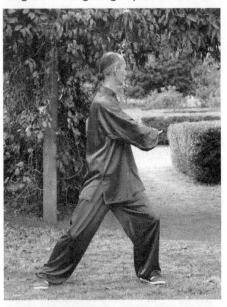

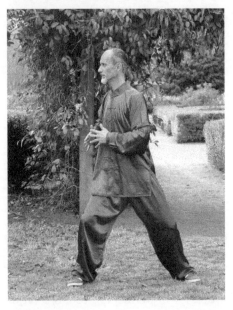

3 Repeat the movement to the left side several times.

BELT MERIDIAN GRINDING

4 Change direction describing a small horizontal S-shape movement with the hands out to the right side and in to the left side.

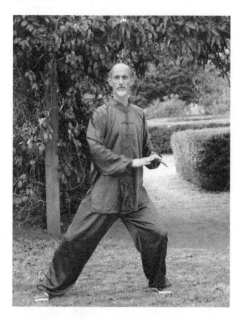

5 Turning from the waist, rotate the hands out to the right side, describing a small horizontal circle toward the right ribs. At the same time shift the weight to the right leg as you breathe in.

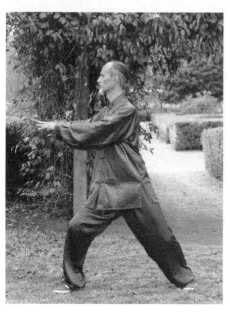

6 In a continuous movement rotate the hands in toward the right ribs, then turning from the waist rotate the hands back to the left side. At the same time shift the weight to the left leg as you breathe out.

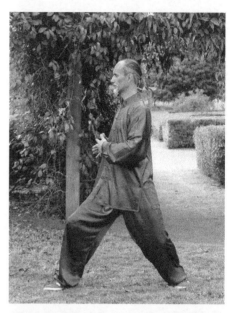

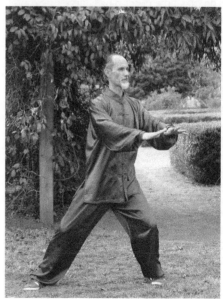

7 Repeat the movement to the right side several times.

BELT MERIDIAN GRINDING

8 Change direction describing a small horizontal S-shape movement with your hands out to the left side and in to the right side.

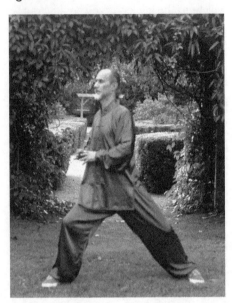

9 Repeat the movement out to the left side, this time describing a large horizontal circle with the hands turning all the way to the back. At the same time shift the weight to the left leg as you breathe in.

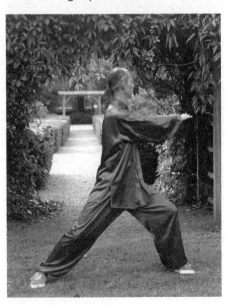

10 In a continuous motion rotate the hands in toward the left ribs, then turning from the waist rotate the hands to the right side. At the same time shift the weight to the right leg as you breathe out.

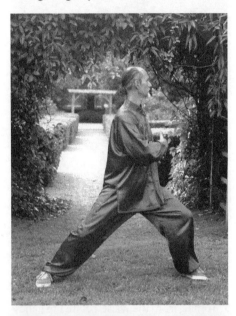

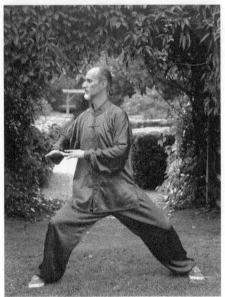

BELT MERIDIAN GRINDING

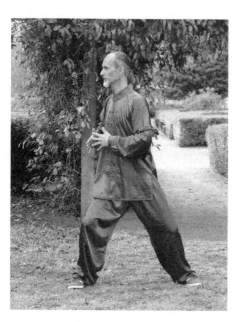

11 Repeat the large horizontal circle out to the left side several times.

12 Change direction describing a small horizontal S-shape movement with the hands out to the right side and in to the left side.

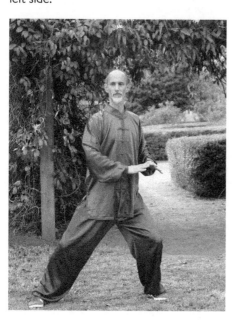

13 Repeat the large horizontal circle out to the right side several times.

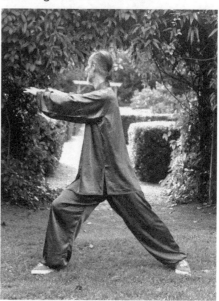

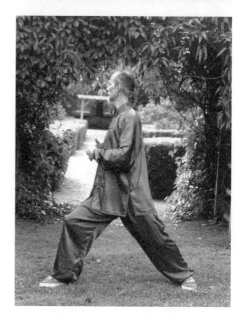

BELT MERIDIAN GRINDING

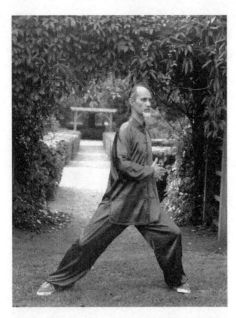

14 End the exercise by bringing the hands to the lower *Dantian*.

Observations

▸ Make sure to turn from the waist and not just from the shoulders or hands.

▸ Keep the hands along a horizontal plane and level with the waist.

▸ Maintain the shoulders lowered and wrist relaxed.

▸ Keep the arms at the height of the waist when turning the body and avoid raising the shoulders.

▸ Keep the knees bent and the heels flat throughout the exercise.

Breathing method

Breathe in when rotating the hands out at the sides. Breathe out when bringing the hands in and back.

Flow of Qi

When the body turns left, Qi moves from left to right around the waist; and when the body turns right, Qi flows from right to left around the waist. Qi circulates in opposite directions around the front and back sides of the waist at the same time.

Mind focus

Focus on turning from the waist and not from the arms, relaxing the waist area, the sensation of Qi flowing as silk around the waist, and coordinating the upper and lower body.

Main Qi channels

Gall bladder, girdle vessel (*Dai Mai*), liver, Yang linking vessel (*Yang Wei Mai*).

Secondary Qi channels

Kidney, large intestine.

Main benefits

▸ Helps to loosen up the waist and the lower back.

▸ Promotes liver and gall bladder functions.

▸ Activates the flow of Qi throughout the body.

▸ Relieves pain in the ribs and hypochondriac region, lower back pain, abdominal bloating, tightness of the chest, stiffness of the neck, shoulders, and back, fibromyalgia, and chronic muscle pain.

▸ Exercises the abdomen and stimulates bowel movement.

▸ Strengthens the kidney Qi.

▸ Tones up the waist and abdomen.

▸ Alleviates symptoms of irregular menses, lower abdominal pain, and hormonal disorders.

PALMS TO EARTH AND SKY

Main vital points

Pericardium 8 (labored palace) on the palm of the hand between the second and third metacarpal bones, Gall Bladder 26 (girdle vessel) on the side of the waist in line with the navel and below the eleventh rib, Stomach 25 (celestial pivot) two inches lateral to the navel, Gall Bladder 22 (armpit abyss) three inches below the center of the armpit, Gall Bladder 23 (sinew seat) one inch anterior to Gall Bladder 22, Gall Bladder 30 (jumping round) on the hip joint, Gall Bladder 34 (Yang mound spring) on the lower leg below the head of the fibula.

Main muscle groups

Anterior deltoid (anterior aspect of shoulder between lateral collar bone and upper arm), pectoralis major (chest region from chest bone and medial collar bone to upper arm), posterior deltoid (posterior aspect of shoulder between shoulder blade and upper arm), teres major (from inferior angle of shoulder blade to medial aspect of upper arm), teres minor (lateral inferior aspect of shoulder blade), latissimus dorsi (from crest of hip bone, sacrum, and lower thoracic vertebrae across middle and lower back to posterior aspect of upper arm), supraspinatus (superior aspect of shoulder blade), pectoralis minor (chest region between anterior 3, 4, and 5 ribs and anterior shoulder blade), extensor carpi radialis brevis (posterior aspect of forearm between lateral aspect of elbow and base of third finger), **external oblique** (lateral aspect of abdomen between lower 8 ribs and abdomen), **internal oblique** (lateral aspect of abdomen from anterior hip bone to lower 4 ribs and abdomen), transversospinalis (along back between transverse processes and spinous processes of vertebrae), **rotators** (between transverse processes and spinous processes of vertebrae), sternocleidomastoid (anterior lateral aspect of neck from superior chest bone and medial collar bone to mastoid bone behind ear), gluteus maximus (buttock area from hip bone to lateral aspect of thigh), popliteus (posterior aspect of knee).

Secondary muscle groups

Serratus anterior (chest wall between upper 8 ribs and anterior surface of shoulder blade), rhomboids (shoulder blade area from thoracic vertebrae to medial border of shoulder blade), upper trapezius (neck and shoulder region between neck vertebrae and lateral aspect of collar bone), **scalene anterior** (from cervical vertebrae of C3–C6 to first rib), lower trapezius (middle back between thoracic vertebrae and root of spine of shoulder blade), **gluteus medius** (buttock area from crest of hip bone to head of thigh bone), piriformis (buttock region from sacrum to upper thigh bone), iliacus (pelvic region from inner surface of hip bone to medial superior aspect of thigh bone).

Starting position

Stand with the feet apart twice the width of the shoulders, knees bent, and the palms facing down in front of the lower abdomen.

PALMS TO EARTH AND SKY

Description of the exercise

1 Moving from the waist, rotate the hands to the left side with the palms down facing the earth. At the same time transfer the weight to the left leg as you breathe out.

3 In a continuous movement rotate the hands down the right side, shifting the weight to the right leg. Then, in a quick motion, twist the body to the left side rotating the left hand down and laterally to the lower back with palm facing out, and the right hand medially and up in front of the forehead with palm out. At the same time transfer the weight to the left leg and look down toward the right heel as you breathe out.

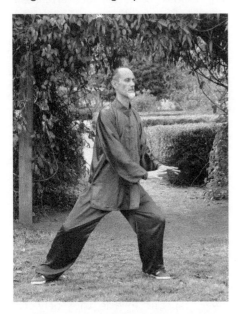

2 Turning from the waist, rotate the hands up the left side and over the head with the palms up facing heaven as you breathe in.

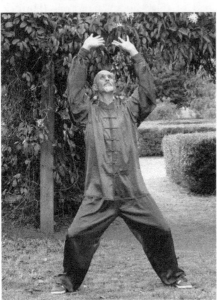

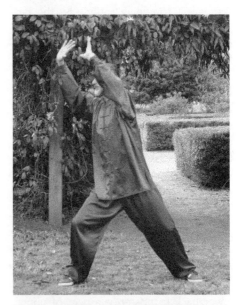

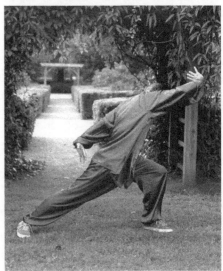

PALMS TO EARTH AND SKY

4 Turn the body to the right side rotating the hands to the right with palms down facing the earth. At the same time transfer the weight to the right leg as you breathe out.

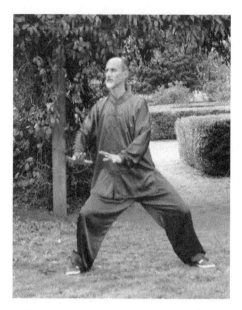

5 Turning from the waist, rotate the hands up the right side and over the head with the palms up facing heaven as you breathe in.

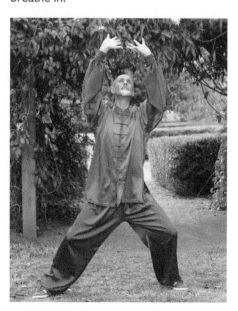

6 In a continuous movement rotate the hands down the left side, shifting the weight to the left leg. Then, in a quick motion, twist the body to the right side rotating the right hand down and laterally to the lower back with palm facing out, and the left hand medially and up in front of the forehead with palm out. At the same time transfer the weight to the right leg and look down to the left heel as you breathe out.

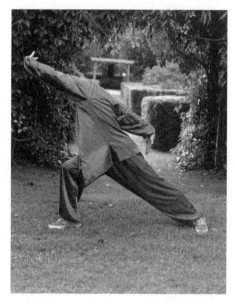

7 Alternate the exercise to the left and right sides several times.

8 End the exercise by bringing the hands to the lower *Dantian*.

Observations

‣ When twisting the body to the sides, align the knee of the weighted leg with the toes.

‣ Turn the body from the waist and not the shoulders.

‣ Keep the shoulders lowered throughout the exercise.

‣ When twisting the body to the sides, look back in the direction of the rear hand.

PALMS TO EARTH AND SKY

Precautions and contraindications

This exercise can be contraindicated in cases of serious back conditions.

Breathing method

Breathe out when turning with the palms facing the earth. Breathe in when turning with the palms facing the sky, and breathe out again when twisting the body.

Flow of Qi

Qi flows from side to side of the waist, and up and down across the back, shoulders, neck, arms, hip and leg.

Mind focus

Focus on turning from the waist, twisting the spine, pushing the hands in opposite directions when twisting the body, and coordinating the upper and lower body.

Main Qi channels

Liver, gall bladder, Yang linking vessel (*Yang Wei Mai*).

Secondary Qi channels

Yin linking vessel (*Yin Wei Mai*), pericardium, three heaters.

Main benefits

- Works out the waist, hips, back, shoulders, and ribs.

- Relieves tightness and pain in the middle back, lower back, shoulders, and neck.

- Helps to stretch the waist and ribs.

- Increases flexibility of the spine.

- Helps to connect the flow of vital energy between the lower and the upper halves of the body.

- Stimulates the flow of gall bladder Qi and liver Qi.

- Activates the Yang linking channel (*Yang Wei Mai*) connecting the flow of Yang Qi throughout the body, and controlling the flow of Qi between the surface and the interior of the body.

- Relieves tightness of the chest, pain in the lateral rib region, tenderness of the breasts, swelling of the armpit, and pain in the hip.

Chapter 15

Daoist Yoga Exercises for the Liver Energy Meridian

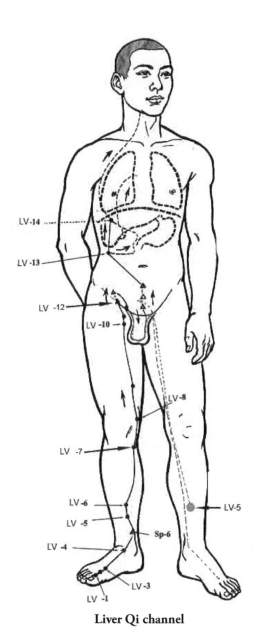

Liver Qi channel

Pathway of the Qi channel

The liver channel starts from the lateral side of the big toe, travels up over the dorsum of the foot between the first and second toes, and moves up anterior to the inner ankle bone. It then runs up the medial aspect of the lower leg, the medial side of the knee, and along the inner midline of the thigh. The channel continues running up along the groin area, the lower abdomen, and the lateral aspect of the trunk to a point inferior to the eleventh free rib. It then moves up over the ribs ending at the sixth intercostal space. The liver channel has 14 vital points.

Internal branches

1. From the upper thigh (Liver 12) a branch goes out to the external genitalia (testes) and enters the lower abdomen.

2. From the lateral aspect of the trunk (Liver 13) an internal branch connects to the stomach, the liver, and the gall bladder.

3. From the space between the sixth and seventh ribs (Liver 14) a branch moves up passing through the diaphragm, hypochondriac region, chest, posterior aspect of the throat (pharynx), and up the face connecting to the eye system. From the eyes the branch travels up the forehead all the way up to the vertex of the head and connects to the brain (Governing Vessel 20). From the eyes another branch travels down over the cheeks and curves around the inner surface of the lips.

4. The branch from the liver passes through the diaphragm and enters the lungs.

Main signs of imbalance

Signs of excess (Fullness of Qi)

Pain, soreness, and fullness of the lateral rib area (hypochondriac region), fullness and pain of the abdomen, bitter taste in the mouth, vomiting, yellow discoloration of the skin (jaundice), irritability, anger, temporal headaches, migraine, vertigo, redness of the eyes, ringing in the ears with a high pitch (tinnitus), high blood pressure, swelling of the thyroid, thyroid nodules, sensation of a lump in the throat, frequent sighing, tenderness of the breast, lumps in the breast, breast fibroids, mood swings, alternation of anger and depression, irregular menses, painful periods, lower abdominal pain, heavy periods with red bright color, premenstrual syndrome (PMS), uterine fibroids, tightness of the mid-back, shoulder blades, and neck area, swelling and pain of the testicles, difficult urination, and excessive sexual desire.

Signs of weakness (Emptiness of Qi)

Blurry vision, night blindness, floaters or dark spots on the visual field, dry eyes, light dizziness, nervousness, tics, low spirit, irritability, mild depression, fatigue, tendency toward constipation, generalized stiffness and tightness of the muscles, chronic muscle pain, scanty menstrual flow, lack of menses (amenorrhea), and severe itching of the skin.

Main areas covered

Big toe, dorsum of foot between second and third toes, medial aspect of lower leg, medial aspect of knee, midline of inner thigh, groin area, reproductive system, rib area, hypochondriac region, liver, gall bladder, stomach, diaphragm, chest, esophagus, pharynx, throat, eyes, brain, vertex of head, and inner lips.

SOOTHING THE FLOW OF LIVER QI

Main vital points

Pericardium 8 (labored palace) on the center of the palm between the second and third metacarpal bones, Pericardium 9 (central hub) at the center of the tip of the middle finger, Liver 13 (bright gate) on the sides of the abdomen just inferior to the eleventh rib, Conception Vessel 17 (middle of the breasts) on the center of the chest between the breasts, *Dantian* (elixir field) on the lower abdomen one third the distance between the navel and the pubic bone.

Main muscle groups

Extensor carpi radialis brevis (posterior aspect of forearm between lateral aspect of elbow and base of third finger), **biceps brachii** (anterior aspect of upper arm), **brachialis** (anterior inferior aspect of upper arm between upper arm bone and ulna bone), pectoralis minor (chest area between anterior 3, 4, and 5 ribs and superior aspect of shoulder blade), serratus anterior (chest wall between upper 8 ribs and anterior surface of shoulder blade), **rhomboids** (shoulder blade area from thoracic vertebrae to medial border of shoulder blade), middle trapezius (upper back area from thoracic vertebrae to spine of shoulder blade), middle deltoid (lateral superior aspect of upper arm), posterior deltoid (posterior aspect of shoulder between shoulder blade and upper arm), **anterior deltoid** (anterior aspect of shoulder between lateral collar bone and upper arm), pectoralis major (chest region from chest bone and medial collar bone to upper arm), **pronator teres** (anterior aspect of forearm across from medial elbow to middle of lateral radius bone), pronator quadratus (horizontally across proximal aspect of wrist).

Secondary muscle groups

Extensor carpi radialis longus (posterior aspect of forearm between lateral aspect of elbow and base of second finger), extensor carpi ulnaris (posterior aspect of forearm between lateral aspect of elbow and base of fifth finger), supraspinatus (superior aspect of shoulder blade), intercostals (between ribs).

Starting position

Stand with the feet shoulder-width apart, knees slightly bent, and the arms down along the sides of the body.

Description of the exercise

1 Place the hands at the sides of the body with the palms facing down and fingers pointing to the front.

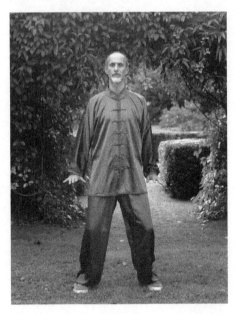

SOOTHING THE FLOW OF LIVER QI

2 Slowly move the hands up the sides of the body along the ribs as you breathe in. Make sure to keep the shoulders lowered.

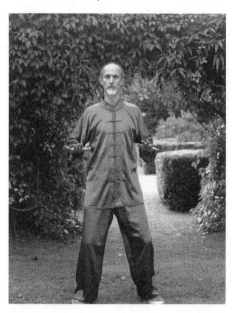

3 Move the hands down along the sides of the body to the waist level, keeping the elbows slightly flexed. At the same time breathe out and drop the body.

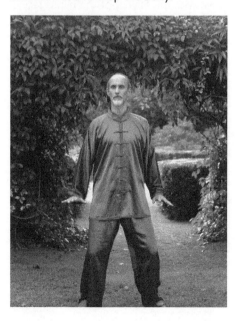

4 Repeat the movement two more times.

5 Bring the hands up to the chest level with the palms facing the front as you breathe in.

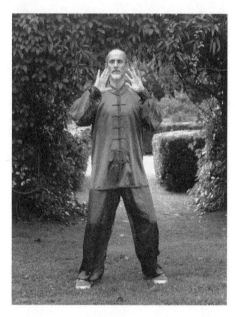

6 From the chest extend the hands in front of the body with the palms facing out as you breathe out. Keep the elbows slightly bent.

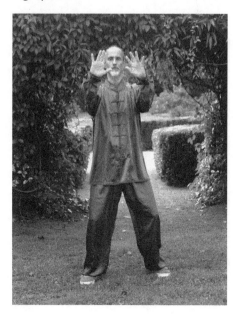

SOOTHING THE FLOW OF LIVER QI

7 Bring the hands back in front of the chest with the palms facing the front as you breathe in.

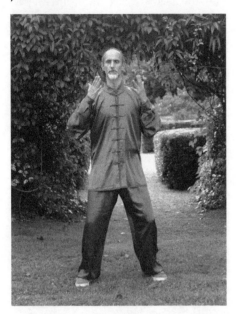

8 Repeat the movement two more times.

9 From the chest extend the hands to the sides of the body turning the palms to face out as you breathe out. Keep a slight bend at the elbows and the shoulders lowered.

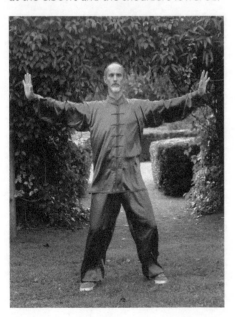

10 Bring the hands back in front of the chest with the palms facing the body as you breathe in.

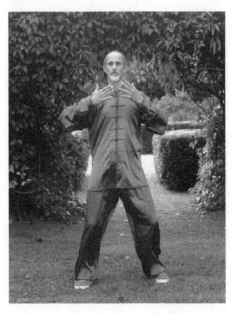

11 Repeat the movement two more times.

12 From the chest turn the palms to face down with the fingers of the hands facing each other.

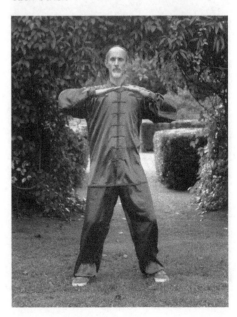

SOOTHING THE FLOW OF LIVER QI

13 Move the palms down the front of the body to the lower *Dantian* center as you breathe out.

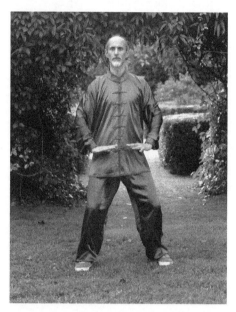

14 Turn the palms up and bring the hands up the front of the body to the chest level as you breathe in.

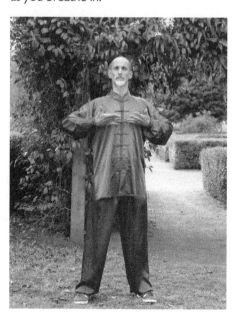

15 Repeat the movement two more times.

16 Repeat the whole set of movements two more times.

17 End the exercise by bringing the hands to the lower *Dantian*.

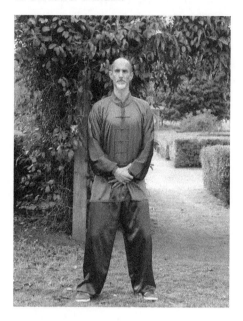

Observations

‣ Keep the shoulders lowered throughout the exercise.

‣ Coordinate the movement of the hands with the breathing.

‣ Maintain the elbows slightly flexed.

Breathing method

Breathe in when moving the hands up or toward the body. Breathe out when moving the hands down and away from the body.

SOOTHING THE FLOW OF LIVER QI

Flow of Qi

From the interior of the body the Qi of the liver spreads upward, forward, sideways, and downward, smoothing out in all directions. Qi also flows along the pericardium energy pathway to the center of the palms and the tip of the middle fingers.

Mind focus

When breathing in, focus on Qi moving to the interior of the body; and when breathing out, focus the mind on the *Lao Gong* cavities located on the center of the palms. At the same time, follow the sensation of Qi reaching the palms and further to the tip of the middle fingers (pericardium channel).

Main Qi channel

Liver.

Secondary Qi channels

Gall bladder, pericardium, lung, heart.

Main benefits

› Helps to decongest the liver and smooth out the flow of liver Qi.

› Improves liver function.

› Stimulates the flow of vital energy or Qi throughout the body.

› Relieves pain in the area below the ribs (hypochondriac region), soreness of the ribs, and tightness of the chest.

› Helps in preventing nervous tension, stress, high blood pressure, dizziness, irritability, tenderness in the breasts, irregular menses, cold limbs, poor digestion, abdominal bloating, and chronic liver disorders.

› Calms the mind and relaxes the nerves.

TURNING RIGHT AND LEFT WITH TWIST

Main vital points

Pericardium 8 (labored palace) on the center of the palm between the second and third metacarpal bones, Gall Bladder 26 (girdle vessel) on the side of the waist level with the navel, Gall Bladder 21 (shoulder well) at the highest point of the shoulder, Liver 13 (bright door) inferior to the eleventh free rib, Urinary Bladder 18 (liver transport) on the mid-back 1.5 inches lateral to the ninth thoracic vertebra, Urinary Bladder 19 (gall bladder transport) on the middle back 1.5 inches lateral to the inferior border of the tenth thoracic vertebra, Gall Bladder 30 (jumping round) on the buttock area just posterior to the hip joint.

Main muscle groups

Biceps brachii (anterior aspect of upper arm), **middle deltoid** (lateral superior aspect of upper arm), supraspinatus (superior aspect of shoulder blade), **posterior deltoid** (posterior aspect of shoulder between shoulder blade and upper arm), **rhomboids** (shoulder blade area from thoracic vertebrae to medial border of shoulder blade), rectus abdominis (anterior aspect of abdomen between pubic bone and lower end of chest bone), **external oblique** (lateral aspect of abdomen from lower 8 ribs to hip bone and abdomen), **internal oblique** (lateral aspect of abdomen from anterior hip bone to lower 4 ribs and abdomen), transverse abdominis (horizontally across abdomen from lower back and ribs to abdomen and pubic bone), **transversospinalis** (along back between transverse processes and spinous processes of vertebrae), **rotators** (from transverse processes of all vertebrae to spinous processes of all vertebrae), pectoralis major (chest region from chest bone and medial collar bone to upper arm).

Secondary muscle groups

Coracobrachialis (anterior medial aspect of upper arm), hamstrings (posterior aspect of thigh between sitting bone and posterior knee), tensor fasciae latae (lateral aspect of thigh between hip bone and lateral aspect of knee).

Starting position

Stand with the feet apart twice the width of the shoulders, knees bent, and hands by the rib sides with palms facing up.

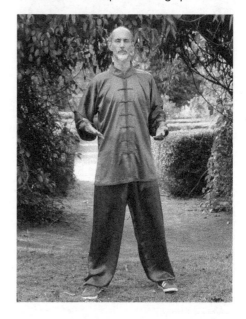

TURNING RIGHT AND LEFT WITH TWIST

Description of the exercise

I Shift the weight to the left leg extending the left hand out from the side of the left ribs as you breathe out.

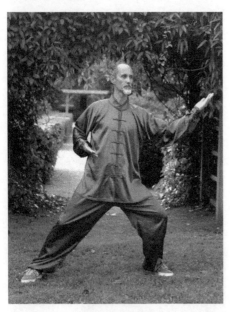

2 Shift the weight to the right leg drawing the left hand toward the body and extending the right hand out from the side of the right ribs as you breathe in.

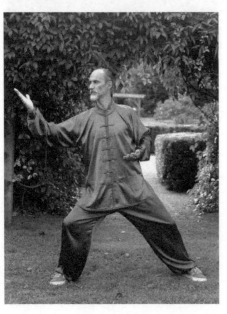

3 Straighten up the body extending the arms out, then twist and bend the body to the left side. At the same time bring the right hand down the outside of the left foot and extend the left hand up the left side as you breathe out. The palms end facing back with the arms straight on a vertical line.

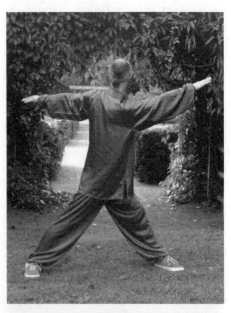

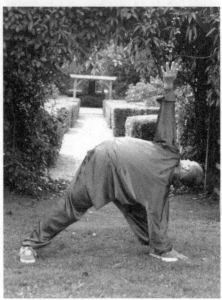

TURNING RIGHT AND LEFT WITH TWIST

4 Straighten up the body and shift the weight to the right leg. At the same time, drawing the left hand toward the body and extending the right hand out from the right ribs as you breathe out.

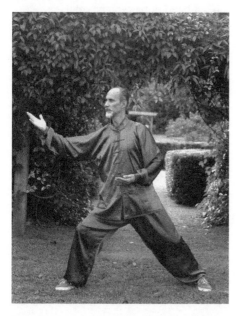

5 Shift the weight to the left leg drawing the right hand in and extending the left hand out from the left ribs as you breathe in.

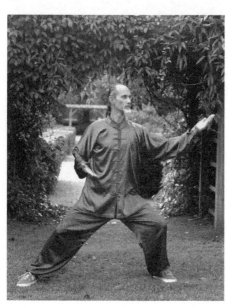

6 Straighten up the body extending the arms out, then twist and bend the body down the right side. At the same time, bring the left hand down the outside of the right foot and extend the right arm up the right side as you breathe out. The palms end facing back with the arms straight on a vertical line.

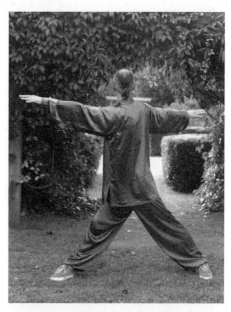

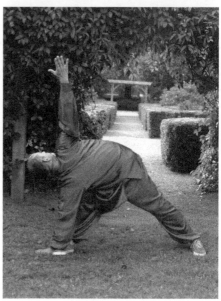

TURNING RIGHT AND LEFT WITH TWIST

7 Repeat twisting and bending the body to the left and right sides several times.

8 In a continuous movement shift the weight to the left leg drawing the right hand in and extending the left hand out from the sides as you breathe in.

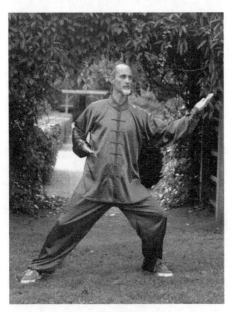

9 Shift the weight to the right leg drawing the left hand in and extending the right hand out from the sides as you breathe out. Again, shift the weight to the left leg drawing the right hand in and extending the left hand out as you breathe in.

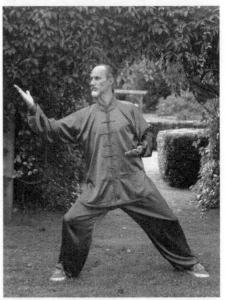

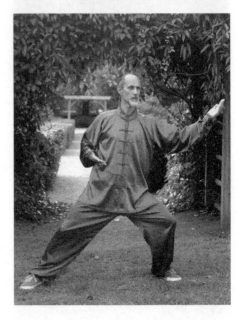

TURNING RIGHT AND LEFT WITH TWIST

10 Straighten the body extending the arms out and turning to the right. Then, in a quick motion, twist and bend the body to the left side as you breathe out. At the same time, bring the right hand down the side of the left foot, and extend the left hand up the left side with palms facing back.

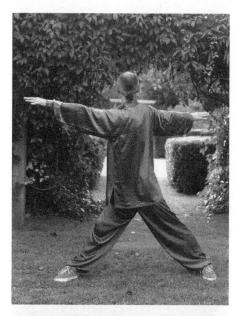

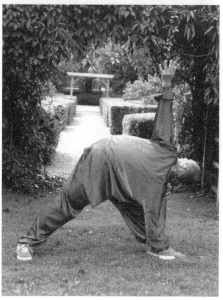

11 Straighten up the body and shift the weight to the right leg. At the same time, drawing in the left hand and extending the right hand out from the ribs as you breathe in.

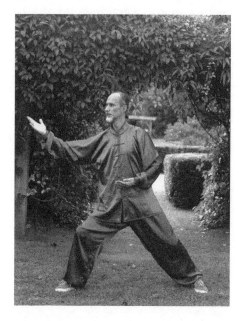

TURNING RIGHT AND LEFT WITH TWIST

12 Shift the weight to the left leg drawing the right hand in and extending the left hand out from the ribs as you breathe out. Again, shift the weight to the right leg drawing the left hand in and extending the right hand out from the ribs as you breathe in.

13 Straighten the body extending the arms out and turning to the left. Then, in a quick motion, twist and bend to the right side as you breathe out. At the same time bring the left hand down the side of the right foot and extend the right hand up the right side with palms facing back.

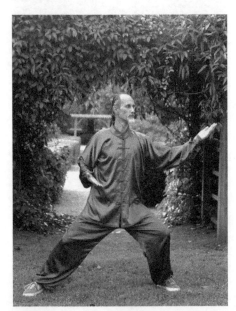

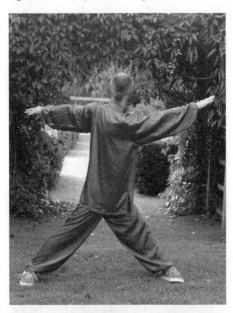

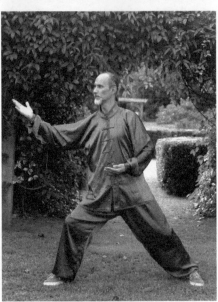

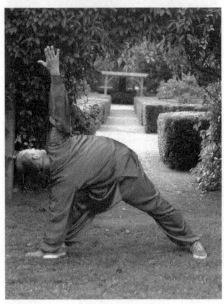

TURNING RIGHT AND LEFT WITH TWIST

14 Repeat twisting and bending the body to the left and right sides several times.

15 End the exercise by straightening up the body and bringing the hands to the lower *Dantian*.

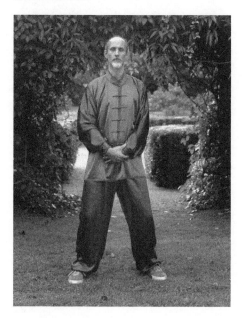

Observations

‣ Straighten the body before turning, bending, and twisting.

‣ Keep shoulders lowered and relaxed.

‣ When turning and twisting the body, maintain the arms in a straight line.

‣ Coordinate the movements of the body with the breathing.

Precautions and contraindications

This exercise may be contraindicated in cases of slipped lumbar disc, sciatica, serious back conditions, hernias, high blood pressure, and vertigo.

Breathing method

Breathe in when straightening the body and breathe out when bending and twisting the body. The specific breathing method is described above in the explanation of the exercise.

Flow of Qi

Qi flows out to the rib sides then across the abdomen and ribs to the middle back, chest, shoulders, and arms. When bending and twisting the body, Qi also flows down the leg.

Mind focus

Focus on the flow of Qi along the rib sides, extending the arms and straightening the body before turning, twisting, and bending down, and alternately compressing and extending the rib sides and abdomen.

Main Qi channels

Liver, gall bladder.

Secondary Qi channels

Girdle vessel (*Dai Mai*), spleen, large intestine, three heaters.

Main benefits

‣ Increases flexibility of the hip, middle back, shoulders, and neck muscles.

‣ Releases congestion of the liver Qi, promoting liver function.

‣ Alternately compresses and stretches the abdomen and rib region massaging the abdominal organs including the liver, gall bladder, pancreas, and spleen.

‣ Improves digestion, stimulates intestinal movement, and relieves constipation.

‣ Opens up the spine and tones the back nerves, stimulating energy flow throughout the body.

‣ Helps to alleviate depression.

‣ Relieves hip and lower back pain.

‣ Helps in reducing the waist line.

‣ Activates the flow of Qi or vital energy along the liver and gall bladder channels.

GLOSSARY

C

Chong Mai: Thrusting vessel

Circadian: Twenty-four hour cycle

D

Dai Mai: Girdle or belt vessel

Dantian: Field of elixir; primary energy center located in the lower abdomen and lower back

Daoyin: Leading and guiding Qi; ancient form of *Qigong*

Dong: Active, movement

Du Mai: Governing or controlling vessel

H

Hatha yoga: Literally, union of sun and moon; traditional yoga system directed to achieve the union of the vital and mental energies

Huxi Daoyin: Guiding the breath

J

Jing Zheng: Primary Qi channels

Jue Yin: Extreme Yin channel

K

Kanda: Sanskrit term meaning a bulb, root, or center

L

Liu Qi: The six levels or divisions of the Qi channels

M

Ming Men: Life gate

Mu: Alarm points located on the front of the trunk

N

Nadi: Sanskrit term meaning currents or subtle channels of *prana* (life force)

Nei Gong: Internal exercise

P

Prana: Sanskrit term meaning vital life force

Q

Qi: Vital life energy

Qi channels: Pathways for the flow of vital energy; energy meridians

Qi Chen Dantian: Sinking the Qi to the *Dantian* center

Qi Gang: The sensation of Qi

Qigong: The practice and skill of cultivating Qi or life energy

Qing Qi: Clear Qi, air

R

Ren Mai: Conception or function vessel

S

San Tiao: Three adjustments or three regulations

Shao Yang: Lesser or young Yang channel

Shao Yin: Lesser or young Yin channel

Shu: Transport points located on the back of the body

Song (Sung): The skill of relaxation; to let loose, opened and expanded

T

Taiji Quan (Tai Chi Chuan): Literal translation, 'great ultimate fist'; internal martial art system, health and longevity exercise

Tai Yang: Greater Yang Qi channel

Tai Yin: Greater Yin Qi channel

Three heaters: The three main energy spaces of the body: lower abdomen, middle abdomen, and chest

Tiao Xi: Regulating the breathing

W

Wai Gong: External exercise

X

Xing: Posture or frame

Y

Yang Ming: Yang bright Qi channel

Yang Qi: The active and creative aspect of Qi

Yang Qiao Mai: Yang motility vessel

Yang Wei Mai: Yang linking vessel

Yi: Mind intent, focus

Yi Nian Daoyin: Guiding the mind

Yin Qi: The receptive and nurturing aspect of Qi

Yin Wei Mai: Yin linking vessel

Yoga: Sanskrit term meaning union, yoking, or binding together

Yuan Qi: Original or prenatal Qi

Yun Dong Daoyin: Guiding movement

Z

Zhen Qi: True Qi

ABOUT THE AUTHOR

Lao Shi Camilo Sanchez, L.Ac., MOM

With 25 years of clinical and teaching experience in acupuncture and Chinese medicine, Camilo has shared his passion of the Daoist healing arts with thousands of clients throughout the United States and South America.

Camilo is a licensed acupuncturist with a master's degree in Oriental Medicine and a recognized teacher of Taiji and Qigong. His areas of expertise include self-healing, preventative therapies, Qigong consulting, and mind–body wellness.

In 1982 the recognized Himalayan yoga Master Swami Satyananda Paramahansa initiated Camilo into the authentic tradition of yoga while in residence at the Satyananda ashram in Munger, India. He was introduced to the arts of Daoist healing and Taiji in 1986 under the tutelage of Dr. Rev. Richard Browne at the Acupuncture and Massage College in Miami, Florida. Subsequently, Camilo has studied with various notable Qigong and Taiji Masters, both in the United States and abroad, including Master Wang Fengming, Master Chunyi Lin, and Master Shu Dong Li.

Camilo is a 20th generation lineage disciple under 19th generation Chen Taiji Master Zhang Xue Xin. Master Zhang is both a direct student of the late 18th generation Chen Taiji lineage holder Master Chen Zhaokui and top senior disciple of Grand Master Feng Zhiqiang of Beijing.

Camilo received the true tradition of the Tao teachings and Taiji under Master F.J. Paolillo in the tradition of Masters Kay Qi Leung and Li En Jiu, which traces its origins to the Chen family, the source of Taiji practice. His Bagua Zhang training comes through the lineage of Master Hing Lun Kwan.

Camilo is a past faculty member of the Acupuncture and Massage College in Florida and the Atlantic University of Chinese Medicine. He has been featured on national television and on radio speaking on the subjects of Chinese medicine and integrated health.

Camilo is founder and director of the Empower Life Center in Charlotte, North Carolina, where he provides custom-based healing and treatment programs of acupuncture and Chinese medicine, and authentic instruction of Taiji, Qigong, and Daoist yoga. His approach to wellness is guiding and empowering each person to awaken the remarkable healing power of the life energy within.

Camilo can be reached for treatment programs, private instruction, speaking engagements, Qigong health consulting, and seminars at the Empower Life Center in Charlotte, NC.

Contact information
Lao Shi Camilo Sanchez, L.Ac., MOM
Empower Life Center
www.empowerlifecenter.com
info@empowerlifecenter.com
704-542-8088

INDEX

Sub-headings in *italics* indicate tables and figures.